SUPERVISION
IN SPEECH
PATHOLOGY

SUPERVISION IN SPEECH PATHOLOGY
A Handbook for Supervisors and Clinicians

Albert R. Oratio,
Bowling Green State University

University Park Press
Baltimore · London · Tokyo

UNIVERSITY PARK PRESS
International Publishers in Science and Medicine
Chamber of Commerce Building
Baltimore, Maryland 21202

Copyright © 1977 by University Park Press
Typeset by The Composing Room of Michigan, Inc.
Manufactured in the United States of America by The Maple Press
Company

Library of Congress Cataloging in Publication Data
Oratio, Albert R.
Supervision in speech pathology.

1. Speech, Disorders of--Study and teaching.
2. Speech therapy--Study and teaching. I. Title.
RC428.07   616.8'55'06   77-4187
ISBN 0-8391-1113-4

CONTENTS

FIGURES

TABLES

PREFACE

Relevant articles on supervision have appeared annually in major journals and at national conventions. Workshops in supervision are on the increase throughout the country. However, there is a paucity, indeed a complete absence, of a major collection of supervisory research and theory within a single volume. If we are to ever effectively traverse the supervisory terrain, map what is known and what needs to be known, and order our priorities for future exploration, it will be necessary to make a comprehensive collection and study of the research, synthesize theories and principles, and propose unifying models for clinicians and supervisors alike. This is the lofty goal of the present volume.

This handbook reflects current supervisory theory and research within a broad spectrum of the social and behavioral sciences, including the professions of social work, education, psychology, psychiatry, counseling, speech communication, and speech pathology. It is, furthermore, a reflection of the author's personal and professional experiences as both a speech clinician and a clinical supervisor. Indeed, much of what is known about these practices is derived from experience.

This book is intended for use by two groups of professionals, supervisors and clinicians. It strives to unite the clinical and supervisory processes into a single, cohesive, conceptual framework. Although the term "clinical supervision" has been used liberally throughout the book, the principles, theories, and research presented are not specific to the clinical practicum experience alone. Rather they apply to a broader range of supervisory-clinical training contexts, such as the Clinical Fellowship Year and student teaching experience. In all contexts, clinical supervision is conceptualized as a supportive and specialized function requiring specific skills in designing facilitatory supervisory conditions.

Chapter 1 is an overview which briefly traces the development of supervision in speech pathology from a historical perspective. Chapter 2 offers working definitions, processes, and methods of supervision based on literature in speech pathology. Chapter 3 is intended specifically for the speech clinician and attempts to capture the essence of the training experience from multiple perspectives. It also provides a comprehensive review of research on interactive methodology. Chapter 4 attempts to synthesize the complex interplay of interaction between supervisor and clinician during the process of clinical training. Chapter 5 deals with the implications of counseling theory for supervision and applies this theory to a method of supervisory interaction analysis. Chapter 6 represents a comprehensive and integrated model of the supervisory process. It calls for specialized training of supervisors and the ability to devote rigorous energy to an intensive cycle of clinical training. Furthermore, it challenges the notion of whether supervision in speech pathology will remain a "stepchild in training."

ACKNOWLEDGMENTS

Although I am grateful to many of my colleagues who have contributed to this work, I am particularly indebted to the following people for providing assistance during the preparation of this book.

I first owe thanks to Dr. Gerard Caracciolo who, during my inception into speech pathology, introduced me to the clinical-supervisory paradigm. He understands the mystery of these processes—his influence is apparent throughout this volume. Appreciation is due Dr. Melvin Hyman, who for the past two years supported and encouraged my interest and pursuit of the area of clinical supervision. My gratitude is also expressed to Dr. John Johnson, for the opportunity to write this book and for his stubborn refusal to let my ideas pass unchallenged. Without him there would be no book. My colleague and close companion, Dr. William O. Haynes, helped spark my efforts and provided the impetus for this writing. For his evaluation and encouragement I am truly indebted. My deepest respect goes to Dr. Harold Henderson, who during this writing stirred my thoughts, nurtured my ideas, and freed me to find my own best way. I gratefully acknowledge the generous evaluation and powerful inspiration received by my former teacher and very special mentor, Dr. Elaine Barden. Her impact has been pervasive. I owe thanks to Dr. Stephen B. Hood, for his red-pencil editing, continued support, and sound advice. His determination and interest in this area helped spur me on. A great deal of appreciation is due Janet Watson, whose careful proofreading, insurmountable patience, and typing skill are unsurpassed. Finally, a special kind of debt is owed to my wife and personal supervisor, Suzanne. She has helped more than words can describe.

To my student clinicians,
from whom I have learned as much as I have taught,
this book is dedicated with admiration.

SUPERVISION IN SPEECH PATHOLOGY

As awareness of the importance of supervision heightens, and as research into supervisory and clinical processes continues, the training of speech clinicians and the profession of speech pathology profit.

chapter 1

INTRODUCTION AND OVERVIEW OF CLINICAL SUPERVISION

During the past 15 years, the concept of supervision has grown in popularity and interest within the field of speech pathology. Nuttall (1960) was one of the first to call attention to clinical training by emphasizing the importance of thorough academic preparation prior to clinical practice. His comments were followed by Perkins (1962), who discussed limitatons of supervising student clinicians. For approximately the next 10 years, a steady stream of articles in support of the importance of supervision appeared in the literature. During this time there also appeared a series of articles (Halfond, 1964; Van Riper, 1965; Ward and Webster, 1965a, b) that were concerned with the interstitial aspects of supervision: the fact that supervision serves in the transition of academic preparation and professional practice and functions to transmit skills in practice from master practitioner to student practitioner. Many of these articles emphasized procedures for transmitting clinical skills to students.

During the latter part of the 1960's and early 1970's, a number of surveys of clinical supervisors were conducted in

1

order to assess the need for a specialized form of supervisory training. Influenced by these reports, associations for clinical supervisors have been organized throughout the 1970's in various parts of the country, such as the Council of Michigan Supervisors of Clinical Practicians, the Inter-University Council of Speech and Hearing Supervisors, and the Council of University Supervisors of Practicum in Speech Pathology and Audiology. Systematic investigations into various areas of supervision currently appear more frequently within the professional literature and at national conventions, and modern technology, such as videotaping procedures and computer programming, is being readily applied to the analysis of clinical behavior.

As awareness of the importance of supervision heightens, and as research into supervisory and clinical processes continues, the training of speech clinicians and the profession of speech pathology profit. To pursue a better understanding of the importance of supervision, a review of research which supports clinical supervision, and that which indicates a need for a specialized form of supervisory training, are first discussed.

SUPPORT FOR SUPERVISION

The profession of speech pathology and audiology has supported the concept of supervision as a vital component in the training of speech clinicians. Support emanates from conferences held throughout the country, such as the Highland Park Conference on Graduate Education in Speech Pathology and Audiology (1963), the Conference on Supervision of Speech and Hearing Programs in the Schools (Indiana University, 1966, 1969), the Seminar on Guidelines for Supervision of Clinical Practicum (Boulder, Colorado, 1964), and the American Speech and Hearing Association Task Force on Supervision (1972). The following is a representative citation of the recognized importance of clinical supervision (Villarreal, 1964):

> Clinical practicum is a critical part of the total preparation of one who would prepare himself for the evaluation and alleviation of speech and hearing disorders. Before knowledge learned from books and classroom lectures can be put to use, a considerable degree of clinical competence must be developed. For this, the speech pathologist or audiologist must practice with people. And he must practice under careful supervision until there is no doubt that he can work independently (p. 1).

Further support is reflected in authoritative statements. In 1964 Halfond wrote:

> Of particular concern is the supervisory process, since it appears to be one of the more crucial aspects of professional education (p. 441).

And in discussing the training program at Western Michigan University, Van Riper (1965) stated: "We view the role of the clinical supervisor as one of the most important of all staff functions . . ." (p. 75). Thus, since the middle of the 1960's, the value and importance of supervision has been well recognized within the field of speech pathology.

NEED FOR SPECIALIZED TRAINING IN SUPERVISION

At the same time that the importance of supervision became recognized, supervision came to be viewed as a specialized function requiring a specialized form of training of supervisory personnel. Such views were held during the American Speech and Hearing Association conference on Guidelines for the Internship Year (Kleffner, 1964). Here it was indicated that:

> . . . as a profession we should take steps to develop, improve, and extend our knowledge and skill in the area of clinical supervision.

There is a clear need in speech pathology and audiology for training in supervision (p. 3).

And in the same year, Halfond (1964) wrote:

While we attempt to upgrade the profession, we do not require special competence and training of our supervisory personnel. . . . Supervision is an involved task but it is basic to good clinical training. We must examine supervisory philosophies, training procedures for supervisors and supervisees, and subsequently, we must continue to work to improve this portion of our teaching (p. 441).

These statements were followed by a series of surveys of clinical supervisors working in universities, public schools, and private facilities. One of the early surveys was conducted by Stace and Drexler (1969), who inquired into the amount of training supervisors had who were employed in a variety of settings: private speech and hearing centers including hospital clinics, comprehensive rehabilitation centers, and public health centers. A total of 122 questionnaires were returned which indicated that: 1) a minute percentage of the private centers surveyed had supervisors who received special training; 2) the majority of these centers indicated that special preparation for supervisors was necessary; and 3) the conception of special preparation, although unclear, seemed to be related to the interpersonal aspects of working with people.

Anderson (1972) surveyed 211 public school and university supervisors. A total of 27 percent of the full time and 22 percent of the part time supervisors indicated having had no course work of any kind in the area of supervision. A total of 95 percent of the full time and 81 percent of the part time supervisors felt a need for some special form of supervisory training. In a later survey of 144 university supervisors of clinical practicum (Anderson, 1973), 33 percent reported having had specialized training in supervision. However, only 53 percent of the programs participating in the survey reported provisions for in-service training for their supervisors.

More recently, Schubert and Aitchison (1975) surveyed a total of 501 supervisors of college and university training programs throughout the country. A total of 64 percent of these supervisors received no specialized course work in supervision. Eighteen percent indicated having had one to three semester hours of course work, and 83 percent thought specialized course work in the area of supervision was important. A series of other reports have discussed weaknesses in supervisory procedures in university settings (Falck, 1972; Culatta, Colucci, and Wiggins, 1975), hospitals and clinics (Culatta and Seltzer, 1976), and public school settings (Rees and Smith, 1967, 1968).

Together, these surveys clearly illustrate the lack of training supervisors have received and the need for training in the specialized job functions they must realize. At a time when over 44,000 students are being trained for careers in communicative disorders (Willis and Willis, 1974), this need has become acute!

Within these few pages, an attempt has been made to trace some of the changes in supervisory literature over the past 15 years and to highlight the importance of supervision and the need for specialized training in this area. It is time now to probe more deeply and explore some concepts and methods of supervision within speech pathology.

REFERENCES CITED

Anderson, J. L., Status of supervision in speech, hearing, and language programs in the schools. J. Lang. Speech Hear. Serv. Schools, 3, 12–23 (1972).

Anderson, J. L., Status of college and university programs of practicum in the schools. Asha, 15, 60–68 (1973).

Culatta, R., Colucci, S., and Wiggins, E., Clinical supervisors and trainees: Two views of a process. Asha, 17, 152–157 (1975).

Culatta, R., and Seltzer, H., Content and sequence analysis of the supervisory session. Asha, 18, 8–12 (1976).

Falck, V., The role and function of university training programs. Asha, 14, 307–310 (1972).

Halfond, M., Clinical supervision—stepchild in training. Asha, 6, 441–444 (1964).

Kleffner, F., Seminar on guidelines for the internship year. Washington, D.C.: American Speech and Hearing Association (1964).

Nuttall, E. C., When should clinical practice begin? Asha, 6, 207–208 (1960).

Perkins, W., Our profession—What is it? Asha, 4, 339–344 (1962).

Rees, M., and Smith, G., Supervised school experience for student clinicians. Asha, 9, 251–257 (1967).

Rees, M., and Smith, G., Some recommendations for supervised school experiences for student clinicians. Asha, 10, 93–103 (1968).

Schubert, G., and Aitchison, C., A profile of clinical supervisors in college and university speech and hearing training programs. Asha, 17, 440–447 (1975).

Stace, A., and Drexler, A., Special training for supervisors of student clinicians: What private speech and hearing centers do and think about training their supervisors. Asha, 11, 318–320 (1969).

Van Riper, C., Supervision of clinical practice. Asha, 3, 75–77 (1965).

Villarreal, J., Seminar on guidelines for supervision of clinical practicum. Washington, D.C.: American Speech and Hearing Association (1964).

Ward, L., and Webster, E., The training of clinical personnel: I. Issues in conceptualization. Asha, 7, 38–40 (1965a).

Ward, L., and Webster, E., The training of clinical personnel: II. A concept of clinical preparation. Asha, 7, 103–106 (1965b).

Willis, C. R., and Willis, J. B., Survey of training programs in speech pathology and audiology. Asha, 16, 200–202 (1974).

The so-called "objective facts" of speech therapy are not accepted objectively by the clinician; rather, they elicit a subjective, emotional reaction. It is doubtful, therefore, that a purely rational supervisory approach can be effective in a situation in which the clinician is ego involved.

chapter 2

SUPERVISORY CONCEPTS, PARADIGM, AND METHODS

Within the supervisory literature in speech pathology three major concepts recur and cut across the various theoretical approaches. These concepts include the *function, structure,* and *process* of clinical supervision. A major portion of supervisory literature can be classified somewhere within this analytic framework.

Function refers to the operations or tasks of the clinical supervisor, including his* responsibilities and, more specifically, the people or agency to whom he is responsible. *Structure* implies the arrangement of supervisory functions or operations. The structure of clinical supervision, then, follows from its function, so that structure and function become linked together. The third concept, *process,* refers to the dynamic interaction of participants—supervisor, clinician, and client—within the parameters of structure and function.

---

*Masculine pronouns are used throughout the book for the sake of grammatical uniformity and simplicity. They are not meant to be preferential or discriminatory.

The concept of a dynamic process is important because supervision in speech pathology is the kind which involves movement and change, as opposed to a more static supervisory model. The clinical supervisor is, indeed, an agent of change. There is a fourth concept, *supervisory objectives,* which is of primary importance and links all three of the above components. Supervisory objectives are determinative of function, structure, and process and therefore demand specification.

Throughout the following chapters an attempt is made to integrate these major concepts into a functional, unified whole. This chapter deals with supervisory functions, supervisory objectives, three divergent supervisory processes, and the structure of supervisory-therapeutic interaction. Chapter 6 focuses on the arrangement of these major concepts into an holistic, dynamic model of clinical supervision.

SUPERVISORY FUNCTIONS

The supervisor is charged with helping the student develop optimal clinical skill. Although this appears to be a simple statement of supervisory function, the operations of the clinical supervisor are highly dynamic, synergistic, overlapping, and complex. The numerous responsibilities to demonstrate, plan, evaluate, supervise across pathologies, and discharge a host of administrative and clerical tasks, complicate providing an accurate and consistent job description for the clinical supervisor. In recognition of these multifaceted operations, Anderson (1973) delineated some major supervisory functions as consisting of teaching, leadership, evaluation, management, facilitation, analysis, interpersonal relationships, and communication, across employment settings (Figure 1).

Adding to this core of functions is the fact that the supervisor is entrusted with helping to establish directions,

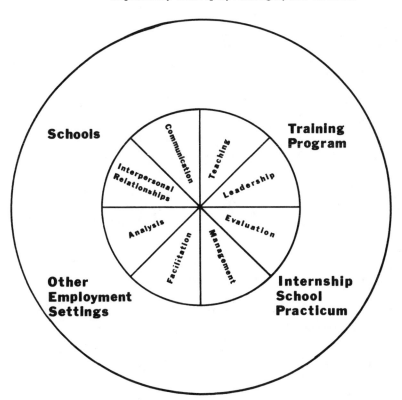

Figure 1. Core supervisory functions. (From Anderson, 1973, p. 13; reprinted with permission.)

goals, and priorities. He assists and guides clinical endeavors. He takes responsibility for the direction and performance of both clinician and client, and assumes major responsibility for the therapeutic strategy and remediation.

A fundamental concern of clinical supervision involves the interrelationship of supervisor, clinician, and client. In most employment settings the supervisor is confronted with dual responsibility for fostering the development of both clinician and client. The essential spirit of supervision entails an ethical responsibility for providing optimal conditions for client progress, and a professional responsibility for enhancing clinician growth. The American Speech and Hearing Association (ASHA) summarized the responsibilities of the supervisor in the university training center as threefold: responsibility to the patient, responsibility to the student, and responsibility to the training center (Villarreal, 1964).

Concern with leadership, analysis, interpersonal relationships, techniques, planning, and clinician-client development is essential, since these are variables in a complex process. Each particular function demands specific levels of skill and training. There is a need to study and understand the interaction of supervisory functions both theoretically and in concrete application.

SUPERVISORY OBJECTIVES

Within the supervisory literature in speech pathology, guidelines for the outcomes of clinical supervision and the procedures for reaching them have been vague. There are many reasons for this lack of clear definition. Some include our lack of knowledge and understanding of the therapeutic process, our lack of experimental research in the area of supervision, and an interest in the role of the clinical supervisor which is only recent. In the absence of definitive objectives, Miner (1967) conceived of the following eight components as the major contents of a program of quality supervision:

1. Understanding and utilizing the dynamics of human relationships which promote the growth of the student clinician.
2. Establishing with the student clinician realistic goals that are clearly understood by both student and supervisor.

3. Observing and analyzing the teaching-learning act involved in the therapy procedures.

4. Providing the student with the feedback necessary to enable him to become increasingly self-analytical.

5. Knowing and using a variety of materials, methods, and techniques which are based on sound theory, successful practice, and documented research.

6. Recognizing and setting aside the supervisor's personal prejudices and biases which influence perception and develop rigidity in order that the subjective task of evaluation may become as objective as possible.

7. Challenging and motivating the student clinician to strengthen his clinical competency without the supervisor's assistance.

8. Appreciating the individual differences among student clinicians to such an extent that supervisory programs and practices may be radically altered to suit each student's needs.

These eight components are reducible to two objectives that form the primary, operational objectives of clinical supervision: 1) to effect a change in clinician behavior, which in turn will change client behavior in a more positive direction, and 2) to enable the clinician to become an independent and autonomous professional. In the early stages of clinical practice the student clinician relies upon the supervisor for methods and procedures that can be utilized for noting and changing clinical behaviors. As supervised practice continues, however, it is essential that these procedures be utilized independent of supervisory impetus, thereby enhancing clinician independence-autonomy through self-supervision. The exact nature of the supervisory process is elaborated in later chapters. The point to emphasize here is that, in a field where both supervisory and therapeutic processes are less precisely measurable, these two goals are forwarded as major objectives of clinical supervision.

Since clinical supervision is concerned with effecting behavioral change, employing particular methods and noting their effect, and developing clinical autonomy, it is in itself a specialized kind of teaching. It is essential, therefore, that supervisors contribute materials, methods, ideas, and procedures for the therapeutic intervention. It is indeed necessary but not sufficient for the supervisor to be proficient at analyzing therapy and planning interventions with the clinician. He himself must be a master clinician. More importantly, however, he must adopt methods and procedures for changing clinician behavior and developing clinical independence and autonomy. These procedures require a specialized form of supervisory training. Practical know-how, specialized training, vision, and ideas are all necessary for improving supervision and hence the training of speech clinicians.

SUPERVISORY PROCESS

The supervisory process involves dynamic interaction among its participants. The nature of this interaction has been a point of controversy across the helping professions. Workers in the medical profession, social work, counselor education, as well as speech pathology, have focused attention on this issue (Rogers, 1957; Boehm, 1961; Romans, 1961; Arbuckle, 1964; Fleming and Benedek, 1964; Ward and Webster, 1965a, 1965b; Delaney and Moore, 1966; Kell and Mueller, 1966; Brown, 1967; Haller, 1967; Miner, 1967; Prather, 1967; Safian, 1967). The problem is clearly related to whether the supervisor-supervisee relationship should take a "cognitive-didactic" approach as contrasted with a "counseling-feeling" approach. Advocates of both approaches are concerned with clinical growth and learning, but they view the supervisory process somewhat differently. Within our own profession, the supervisory process has been defined as a combination of both teaching and counseling approaches (Villarreal, 1964):

> The role of an effective supervisor should transcend the mere monitoring of student's clinical activities. It should include the informal teaching of clinical content, the demonstration of clinical techniques, and the mature counseling of the student in relation to his clinical training (p. 14).

Currently, within the field of speech pathology no uniform practice exists among supervisors concerning a supervisory model or process of clinical training. Supervisory practices range from highly permissive to more rigid, structured procedures (Halfond, 1964; Van Riper, 1965; Ward and Webster, 1965a, 1965b; Brown, 1967; Griffith, 1970). Such philosophical differences result in the execution of supervisory procedures that enable the student to see himself in a dependent situation in which he must take advice from an established authority (Halfond, 1964), or in an independent one containing conditions for continued growth and self-actualization (Ward and Webster, 1965a, 1965b).

The fields of psychology, social work, education, and psychiatry have explored and in some instances tested both theoretical and operational models of supervision (Eckstein and Wallerstein, 1958; Finn and Brown, 1959; Dellis and Stone, 1960; Jedd, Kohn, and Shulman, 1962; Boyan and Copeland, 1974). Although supervision in speech pathology has no single, universally accepted conceptualization, a review of the literature reveals the emergence of three divergent supervisory processes. These processes can be classified as "supervisor-centered," "clinician-centered," and "client-centered" (Engnoth, 1973). Together, these three approaches represent the range of supervisory processes currently in use. Each process is based on a philosophy concerning the nature of clinical skill and effectiveness, and from that belief evolves a particular method for facilitating clinician development. Based on the literature, an attempt has been made to appropriately assign methods to each process. Each process is discussed below in its "pure" form, although in practice supervisory processes exist along a continuum ranging from supervisor centered to client centered.

Supervisor-Centered Process

The supervisor-centered process is based in the philosophy that the supervisor possesses the values, knowledge, and skills that are necessary to be an effective clinician. He therefore sets out to make the clinician over in his own image. Within the process the clinician is placed in an apprentice-like position in which he is the recipient of ongoing instruction. In this sense, the supervisor-centered process is conceived of as a modified teaching situation. Here the supervisor is perceived as an authority figure and "expositor" who offers his expertise and carefully structures a series of procedures that together comprise a kind of supervisory curriculum. These procedures are designed to allow the student to engage in a logical, intellectual process of learning about therapy. A first step in the process may involve the use of lesson plans (King, 1965; Van Riper, 1965; Griffing, 1968), which enable the student to think logically about the therapeutic intervention. Frequent demonstration, observation, and critique take place (Halfond, 1964; Van Ripper, 1965; Kunze, 1967; Darley, 1969). Finally, an element of conferencing may be included. The nature of this process essentially consists of three phases: an initial phase in which the supervisor teaches by example; a second phase in which the supervisor and student engage in coordinated planning and the student executes the management of the client under close supervision; and a third phase in which the student assumes primary responsibility for planning and management under minimal supervision (Villarreal, 1964). Throughout each phase the supervisor imparts clinical

and technical advice in an attempt to help the student integrate theory and practice. He controls the training process
through the selection of supervisory procedures and gradually
releases control as the clinician shows increased ability to
handle the therapeutic intervention.

The most noteworthy aspect of the supervisor-centered
process has little to do with procedural aspects, but has much
to do with supervisory interaction dynamics. Such dynamics
are aimed at getting the clinicain to "know" about therapy.
From the student clinician's point of view, learning about
therapy requires internalization of supervisory standards im-
posed from above, recall of subject matter previously presented in texts and course work, and incorporation of this
material into practice. Consequently, supervisory conference
dynamics typically involve either asking the student questions in an almost Socratic-like style, or telling the student
the "correct" response. These questions test the student's
perceptions of the therapeutic encounter and his knowledge
of theory and methodology. They are designed to bring the
student to some awareness of what he knows and needs to
know about therapy. An interesting example of such a situation is provided by Broudy (1963). He uses the illustration in
which Socrates attempted to teach a slave boy a complicated
theorem. After asking various leading questions, Socrates
asked: "Are you prepared to affirm that the double space is
the square of the diagonal?" to which the slave boy responds,
"Certainly, Socrates" (pp. 12–13). The illustration suggests
that the slave boy learned to respond, "Certainly, Socrates,"
rather than actually acquire a knowledge of the complicated
theorem. Since the questions employed by the supervisor in
this process are those to which he already knows the answer,
one may ask, "Then why ask the question?" The reason
"why" is probably to discover whether the student can
repeat the supervisor's predetermined answer. This tests
whether the student can repeat what the supervisor already
knows.

The supervisor-centered process is a "knowing" approach. It stresses the clinician's cognitive, intellective development. Anderson (1974) indicates that a particular danger in such a tutorial approach to supervision involves the notion that the clinician is apt to imitate the supervisor's clinical style and never realize his own unique potentials. This situation is likely to further the student's dependency upon the supervisor and inadvertently result in a lack of self-confidence. Gitterman (1972) found that supervisors who employ this process come to ask themselves, "Why am I compelled to 'teach,' to 'tell,' to 'lecture,' to 'exhort'?" He stated that there are many reasons, a major one being a need to prove to the student that "I know something!" Perhaps the supervisor-centered supervisor comes to sense his affect and struggles to move beyond his own need to teach and instead becomes a skillful and sensitive cooperative agent.

Clinician-Centered Process

The clinicain-centered process is based on the fact that the clinician is faced daily with important human encounters. Since therapy takes place within a human encounter, it is proposed that human interpersonal processes be the larger part of clinical training. Therefore, it is essential that the supervisor provide conditions for growth and self-actualization of the student clinician. Concern is not with knowledge of theories and methods but with the clinician who implements them. The argument forwarded is that a technique can be no better than the clinician employing it. Furthermore, this approach implies that the supervisory process must be much more than a tutorial, didactic arrangement. It must involve procedures which directly facilitate the clinician's self-study, self-discovery, insight, and behavioral change (Ward and Webster, 1965a, 1965b; Brown, 1967). Ward and Webster (1965b) indicate:

As the student applies the principles of human behavior to himself he also can apply them meaningfully to others, including those with disordered speech and hearing and those whom he encounters in his clinical practice situations (p. 105).

This kind of growth model dictates that the so-called "objective facts" of speech therapy are not accepted objectively by the clinician; rather, they elicit a subjective, emotional reaction. It is doubtful, therefore, that a purely rational supervisory approach can be effective in a situation in which the clinician is ego involved. The clinician as a person must be recognized and dealt with through a kind of counseling framework. Brown (1967) states that:

Familiarity with the work of people like Sullivan, Rogers and Fromm is invaluable. Making use of techniques developed by psychologists, the good supervisor will lead the student to self discovery rather than lecturing to him. The person who makes self discoveries learns emotionally as well as intellectually. This is true learning as contrasted to intellectual understanding without real acceptance of the supervisor's points (p. 477).

The clinician-centered process is essentially a "feeling" approach. Advocates of clinician-centered supervision posit a perceptual or phenomenological theory of the supervisory process. Their viewpoint argues that emphasis upon objective data alone is too narrow an approach. An objective approach alone does not adequately deal with the affective reaction of the student. It excludes the kind of data that are crucial to the student clinician's decision making, that is, his own perceptions of himself in the clinical world of so-called objective facts. These perceptions seem to determine choices, decisions, and behavioral change rather than objective facts themselves.

The clinician-centered process is prone to disadvantages as well as advantages. Focusing primarily upon the clinician's personality may lead to emotional constriction and self-con-sciousness. The clinician may tend to become overly preoc-cupied with his own feelings and emotions rather than with the acquisition of technical skills and the incorporation of such skills into his clinical repertoire and ultimately into practice. The process is in danger of confusing the relation-ship between "feeling" and "doing" in much the same way that the supervisor-centered process lacks integration of "knowing" and "feeling." Although the clinician may de-velop insight or knowledge, he is still in need of monitoring his own clinical activities, thereby developing the skill neces-sary to put effective therapy into practice. On the other hand, in favor of the clinician-centered process is the satisfac-tion said to derive from self-discovery. It is proposed that lasting and effective changes in behavior take place when the clinician works through the process of clinical development in his own way and develops personal insight and his own unique clinical style.

The human relationships between supervisor, clinician, and client are critically determinative of clinical growth and development and therapeutic effectiveness. The clinician-cen-tered process focuses on these interpersonal aspects. What is also needed, however, is an opportunity to transfer insight into action within the therapeutic encounter.

Client-Centered Process

As contrasted with the supervisor-centered and clinician-cen-tered processes, the client-centered process is a "doing" ap-proach. This process proposes that clinical effectiveness is enhanced when the clinician can focus intensively upon the behavior of the client and follow the supervisor's lead in fulfilling the objectives that have been established for both clinician and client.

There are basically two approaches to the client-centered process. The first involves an approach to conferencing. Here the supervisor discusses the client's behavior with the clinician rather than discussing the clinician's own clinical behavior (Prather, 1967). The conference is organized around client reaction. The supervisor focuses the clinician's attention on the client's behavior by structuring a series of questions, such as, "Did you notice how the client participated when you were at the mirror?" "Did you notice how well she did when. . .?" Although an element of clinician behavior enters the discussion, it is relatively minor; primary focus is on client behavior. The clinician simply attends to specific goals for the client, the procedures used to achieve these goals, and the effectiveness of the therapy.

A second approach to client-centered supervision takes place directly within the therapeutic encounter. A simple induction loop and hearing aid receiver are employed in combination with behavior modification procedures for continuous monitoring of therapeutic interaction (Brooks and Hannah, 1967; Latas, 1967; Starkweather, 1974). Through a one-way mirror the supervisor focuses intensely upon the behavior of the client and monitors the clinician's behavior through approval, disapproval, or the feeding of instructions through a microphone that leads to a hearing aid receiver worn by the clinician. Throughout therapy, the clinician is directly trained by the supervisor's auditory presence to respond to the client's behavior.

Proponents of this aspect of client-centered supervision (Brooks and Hannah, 1967; Latas, 1967; Starkweather, 1974) suggest that the approach contains four major advantages. First, feedback to the clinician is immediate. Second, feedback is specified in small units of clinical activity. Third, specificity of feedback permits more complete control of the clinician's behavior and hence the client's behavior. The clinician is clearly able to distinguish between the supervisor's judgment of therapeutic from nontherapeutic clinical activity. Fourth, this behavior modification approach permits systematic recording and quantification of client progress.

The client-centered process gives little emphasis to the clinician's knowledge, cognitive processes, affective reactions, or internal feelings; rather, it is centered on client control. There are some major assumptions involved in the process. First is that the supervisor's judgment is perfect and that the supervisor's clinical frame of reference can be effectively transferred through the use of such an approach. Second is that the novice clinician can be conditioned to match the supervisor's expert judgments and that these judgments will generalize to the clinician's independent involvement with future clients. Furthermore, the process assumes that behavioral techniques constitute the greater whole of an effective therapeutic intervention and that as a training approach, the client-centered process will have lasting effects on the clinician's judgment, behavior, and development.

Integrated Process

It is doubtful that any of the foregoing supervisory processes are or could be employed in their pure form, as discussed above. They do serve, however, to illustrate a range of supervisory processes on a continuum. One of the major differentiating aspects of each process is in the interactions employed between supervisor and clinician. A second differentiating feature lies in the procedures employed to enhance the clinician's development. Each of these processes appears to be effective in fostering at least one aspect of the clinician's development: "knowing," "feeling," or "doing." All three of these aspects are essential for effective speech and language therapy, and in the end, the client will judge the clinician by what he "knows," "feels," and "does."

In Chapter 6, a supervisory model is presented that attempts to integrate all three of these aspects of clinical competence. Didactic elements are included in order to help the clinician obtain technical knowledge, or the "knowing" aspects of therapy. A specialized approach to the supervisory conference is forwarded in detail, to enable the supervisor to enhance the clinician's insight and self-exploration, the "feeling" aspects of clinical development. Self-confrontation and micro-therapeutic procedures are introduced to effect behavior change, and thereby enhance the "doing" component of the trainee's development. An integrated supervisory process is a microcosm of helping to facilitate all aspects of clinical development: cognitive, emotional, and experiential. The ultimate challenge of clinical supervision involves helping the clinician to incorporate all of these aspects into a unique clinical self which will make for a powerful approach to his future clinical practice with clients of all types.

TRIADIC PARADIGM

Cognitive, emotional, and experiential elements have been forwarded as major parameters of clinical competence. These elements are conveyed through interactions which are common to both the supervisory and the therapeutic process. In order to develop a deeper understanding of supervision as a triadic interactive process (Tharp and Wetzel, 1969), a schematic conceptualization of supervision and speech therapy is herein presented.

Both supervisory and therapeutic processes are essentially interactive processes involving reciprocal relationships between supervisor, clinician, and client. The triadic paradigm depicted in Figure 2 indicates that each member of the triad is both an initiator and recipient of overt, external interactions (verbal, gestural) as well as internal interactions (feelings, emotions). Since supervision and speech therapy are largely interpersonal transactive processes, there is a degree of universality in the interactions generated between members of the triad. This common core of interactions has implica-

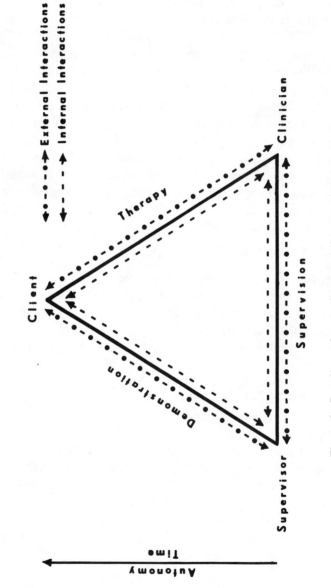

Figure 2. Paradigm of supervisory and therapeutic interaction.

tions for both supervision and speech therapy and contributes to effective or ineffective communications during
these endeavors.

The dual track nature of the paradigm in Figure 2 depicts
transactions on discrete tracks, both internal and external,
for the purpose of simplicity in illustration. However, these
tracks cross and overlap. Overt interactions communicate
feeling tones through eye contact, facial expressions, intona-
tion patterns, and the like, and feelings and emotions gen-
erate and give rise to overt interactions. Some recent research
(Oratio, in preparation) supports this conceptualization of a
strong interrelationship between the interpersonal-emotional
and the technical-gestural aspects of therapeutic behavior.
The relationship between these interactions, therefore, is not
static as illustrated, but dynamic, overlapping, and interrelated. Thus we see that both supervision and speech
therapy are not only verbal communicative processes but also
fundamentally social processes of interaction in which feelings and emotions are generated between members of the
triad.

The structure of the paradigm indicates that the base of
interaction for clinical training is between supervisor and
clinician. This portion is depicted as the supervisory encounter. The therapeutic encounter illustrates the reciproca-
tion of interaction between clinician and client during the
remedial process. Demonstration is illustrated by supervisor-
client transactions. The psychological, interpersonal, social,
and technical exchanges between members of the triad have
their ultimate goal in client autonomy. The structure of these
exchanges is such that, as supervisory and therapeutic processes progress in time, both supervisor and clinician gradually
release client control and thereby encourage higher and more
independent levels of client functioning. Ultimately, transactions must be structured so that the client can monitor and
correct his verbal behavior independent of clinical intervention.

The present model simplifies supervisory reality. The dynamics of the supervisory and therapeutic encounter are highly complex. The interpersonal characterological patterns of each member must always be considered. It is the supervisor who is responsible for recognizing the way in which interpersonal dynamics contribute to both the supervisory and therapeutic processes. Notwithstanding the variety of methods and processes available, both supervision and speech therapy as typically practiced consist of overt verbal-gestural interactions and the exchange of internal feelings and emotions between supervisors, clinicians, and clients. The content and sequence of these exchanges are critical in determining the effectiveness of each process. Research in supervision has concentrated on ways to affect these transactions and thereby improve both supervisory and therapeutic processes.

RESEARCH ON SUPERVISORY METHODOLOGIES

Examination of the supervisory literature in speech pathology indicates that articles pertaining to supervisory methods can be divided into two groups. The first group consists of authoritative suggestions or reports of supervisory methods. These involve reports on general supervisory procedures, including demonstration (King, 1965; Van Riper, 1965; Erickson and Van Riper, 1967), as well as reports on the use of closed circuit television and videotape procedures (O'Neill and Patterson, 1964; Diedrich, 1966). The largest body of research in supervisory methodology falls into the realm of interaction analysis and self-confrontation procedures. Since these procedures constitute important clinician as well as supervisory techniques, they are discussed in the following chapter under interaction analysis.

The second group of studies are systematic attempts to explore a broad range of supervisory procedures and their effects on the training of speech clinicians. One of the first systematic studies was by Ingram and Stunden (1967), who investigated students' attitudes toward the therapeutic process. A total of 120 students were divided into five groups based on educational level and major field of study. Each subject completed a semantic differential containing eight stimulus words that were thought to be related to speech therapy (for example, empathy, rapport, motivation, acceptance). These words were used to assess the student's attitude concerning therapy as a function of training and experience. Findings indicated that graduate and trained undergraduate majors in speech pathology defined the stimulus words more extremely than the other groups, suggesting that the stimulus words have more meaning for these subjects. Since these students showed a heightened sensitivity to words associated with clinical concepts, the authors concluded that training results in a point of view about therapy that is related to the nature of the training task.

In an attempt to investigate supervisors' and clinicians' views of the supervisory process, Culatta, Colucci, and Wiggins (1975) interviewed 36 graduate students and 18 supervisors. Reactions were solicited from subjects concerning report writing, supervisory interaction, therapeutic strategies, use of self-confrontation procedures, conferencing, and evaluation. Sharply differing perceptions between supervisors and clinicians were found to exist in relation to written reports, supervisory interaction, and supervisory evaluation. Clinicians reported uncertainty concerning how their clinical behaviors were evaluated. They further reported a lack of lesson plan requirements and a lack of initial supervisory conferencing. Generally, this study illustrated the need for supervisors and clinicians to develop a mutual understanding of the procedures and methods employed in supervision.

Through the use of filmed therapy sessions, Irwin and Nickles (1970) developed a tool for measuring supervisory judgments of clinician behavior. In that same year, Hall

(1970) investigated the effects of four supervisory conditions on perceived therapeutic effectiveness. Supervisory conditions consisted of the following: 1) no evaluation of clinical performance, 2) videotape replay of clinical performance, 3) conferencing plus evaluation, and 4) conferencing plus videotaping. No significant differences were found between any of the supervisory conditions. An interaction effect for individual clinicians led Hall to conclude that individual differences exist among beginning clinicians that make them respond differently to various forms of supervision.

In a similar study, utilizing a single subject's design, Engnoth (1973) investigated the effects of three supervisory approaches on undergraduate clinicians' degree of behavioral change. Supervisory approaches included: 1) an instructional conference approach, consisting of continual guidance and frequent instruction, direct observation, critique, and weekly conferences; 2) loop supervision, whereby the clinician received immediate feedback (yes, good, no, and so on) through an electronic induction loop system and hearing aid receiver (in this approach lesson plans were not required and conferences were not scheduled); and 3) self-learning supervision, in which the subject received no direct supervision at all. Findings indicated that the clinicians' behavior changed in association with all three supervisory approaches. The subject in the self-learning supervisory approach showed the greatest net change in clinical behavior. All subjects reported a preference for a modified instructional conference type of supervision.

Kaplan and Dreyer (1974) investigated the effect of "self-awareness" training on student clinicians' interpersonal relationships with their clients during therapy. Their findings indicated that subjects receiving training in self-awareness were more socially supportive, used more positive facial and gestural responses, and were less restrictive in therapy than the control group subjects. In addition, the therapeutic climate was more positive, and clients of the experimental group subjects were more cooperative than clients of the control group subjects. The authors concluded that there is support to include self-awareness programs in the training of speech clinicians.

In a unique study, Stech et al. (1973) used a factor-analytic procedure to explore the effects of various client behaviors on speech clinicians' perceptions of those behaviors. Their results indicated that a two-way reinforcement pattern between clinician and client exists during the process of speech therapy. For the 85 clinicians who served as subjects in this study, appropriate responses, evidence of motivation, independent learning, and compliance to the clinicians' requests were the most rewarding forms of client behavior. Negative emotional reaction and a poor interpersonal relationship were viewed by clinicians as most punishing. Inappropriate responses and lack of motivation were felt to be mildly punishing client behaviors. Results of this study suggest that training should include methods for bringing reciprocal therapeutic reinforcement to a conscious level of awareness in clinicians.

CONCLUSIONS

Based on these few studies it would be unwise to attempt to draw formal conclusions. Results of the above studies are, therefore, reviewed cautiously, and four tentative implications are cited below.

First, training in the field of speech pathology seems to take effect as early as the middle portion of undergraduate preparation. Speech pathology majors, at that point in their education, react to concepts germaine to the profession. Second, there appears to be a need for greater coordination of supervision between clinicians and supervisors. Both supervisors and clinicians appear to have differing perceptions of supervisory requirements and expectations. Third, studies of the effects of specific supervisory approaches on the clinician's performance during therapy have ranged from intensive supervision to no direct supervision. Results of these studies have generally yielded no "significant" difference in clinician behavior. Although behavioral changes have been shown to take place among clinicians within these studies, the effects of specific supervisory procedures on clinician behavior are still unclear. Finally, there appears to be an element of reciprocal reinforcement which takes place between clinician and client during the therapeutic process.

Each of these findings has significance for the supervisory process, and each provides indications for future research. Before attempting to relate these findings to supervision, however, further research is needed.

REFERENCES CITED

Anderson, J. L., Supervision: The neglected component of our profession. In: L. J. Turton (ed.), Proceedings of a Workshop on Supervision in Speech Pathology. Ann Arbor, Mich.: University of Michigan (1973).

Anderson, J., Supervision of the clinical process in speech pathology: Issues and practices. Short course presented at the American Speech and Hearing Association Convention, Las Vegas (1974).

Arbuckle, D. S., Supervision: Learning, not counseling. J. Council Psychol., 11, 90–94 (1964).

Boehm, W., Social work: Science and art. Soc. Serv. Rev., 35, 144–151 (1961).

Boyan, N. J., and Copeland, W. D., A training program for supervisors: Anatomy of an educational development. J. Educ. Res., 18, 100–115 (1974).

Brooks, R. S., and Hannah, E. P., A tool for clinical supervision. J. Speech Hear. Disord., 32, 215–227 (1967).

Broudy, S. H., Historic exemplars of teaching method. In: N. Gage (ed.), Handbook of Research in Teaching Education. Chicago: Rand McNally (1963).

Brown, E. J., A university's approach to improving supervision. Asha, 9, 476–479 (1967).

Culatta, R., Colucci, S., and Wiggins, E., Clinical supervisors and trainees: Two views of a process. Asha, 17, 152–157 (1975).

Darley, F., Clinical training for full-time clinical service: A neglected obligation. Asha, 11, 143–148 (1969).

Delaney, D. L., and Moore, J. C., Student expectations of the role of practicum supervisor. Couns. Educ. Sup., 6, 11–17 (1966).

Dellis, N. P., and Stone, J. K., The Training of Psychotherapists. Baton Rouge: Louisiana University Press (1960).

Diedrich, W. M., Use of videotape in teaching clinical skills. Volta Rev., 644–647 (1966).

Eckstein, R., and Wallerstein, R. S., The Teaching and Learning of Psychotherapy. New York: Basic Books (1958).

Engnoth, G. L., A comparison of three approaches to supervision of speech clinicians in training. Unpublished doctoral dissertation, Lawrence, Kan.: University of Kansas (1973).

Erickson, R., and Van Riper, C., Demonstration therapy in a university training program. Asha, 9, 33–35 (1967).

Finn, M. H. P., and Brown, F., Training for Clinical Psychology. New York: International Universities Press (1959).

Fleming, J., and Benedek, T., Supervision: A method of teaching psychoanalysis. Psychoanal. Q., 33, 71–96 (1964).

Gitterman, A., Comparison of educational models and their influence on supervision. In: F. Kaslow (ed.), Issues in Human Services. San Francisco: Jossey-Bass (1972).

Griffing, B. L., Supervision of instruction: Guiding innovation and change in instruction for deaf children. Volta Rev., 70, 678–684 (1968).

Griffith, F. A., Clinical practicum: A problem with no panacea. Unpublished report by Bureau of Child Research, University of Kansas. Submitted to National Institute of Neurological Diseases and Strokes (1970).

Halfond, M., Clinical supervision—stepchild in training. Asha, 6, 441–444 (1964).

Hall, A. S., The effectiveness of videotape recordings as an adjunct to supervision of clinical practicum by speech pathologists. Unpublished doctoral dissertation, Columbus, Ohio: Ohio State University (1970).

Haller, R., Supervisors' criteria for evaluating students' performance in clinical practicum activities. Asha, 9, 479–481 (1967).

Ingram, D., and Stunden, A., Student's attitudes toward the therapeutic process. Asha, 9, 435–442 (1967).

Irwin, R. B., and Nickles, A., Use of audiovisual films in supervised observation. Asha, 12, 363–367 (1970).

Jedd, J., Kohn, R. E., and Shulman, G. L., Group supervision: A vehicle for professional development. Soc. Work, 7, 96–102 (1962).

Kaplan, N. R., and Dreyer, D. E., The effect of self-awareness training on student speech pathologist-client relationships. J. Commun. Disord., 7, 329–342 (1974).

Kell, B. L., and Mueller, W. J., Impact and Change: A Study of Counseling Relationships. New York: Appleton-Century-Crofts (1966).

King, R., Supervision at a university training center. Speech Teach., 14, 178–180 (1965).

Kunze, L. H., Program for training in behavioral observations. Asha, 9, 473–476 (1967).

Latas, W., Techniques of supervision in a temporal framework. Paper presented at the American Speech and Hearing Association convention, Chicago (1967).

Miner, A., Standard for quality supervision of clinical practicum. Asha, 9, 471–472 (1967).

O'Neill, J. J., and Patterson, H. A., The use of closed circuit television in a clinical speech training program. Asha, 6, 445–447 (1964).

Oratio, A. R., Interrelationship between interpersonal and technical skills of student clinicians in speech therapy. In preparation.

Prather, E. M., An approach to clinical supervision. Asha, 9, 472–473 (1967).

Rogers, C., Training individuals to engage in the therapeutic process. In: C. Strother (ed.), Psychology and Mental Health. Washington, D.C.: American Psychological Association (1957).

Romans, J., Teaching of psychiatry to medical students. Lancet, 93–95 (1961).

Safian, M. Z., The application of psychodynamic principles to the clinical work of the speech and hearing pathologist: Conference summary. J. Commun. Disord., 1, 54–57 (1967).

Starkweather, C. W., Behavior modification in training speech clinicians: Procedures and implications. Asha, 16, 607–611 (1974).

Stech, E. L., Curtiss, J. W., Troesch, P. J., and Binnie, C., Clients' reinforcement of speech clinicians: A factor-analytic study. Asha, 15, 287–289 (1973).

Tharp, R., and Wetzel, R., Behavior Modification in the Natural Environment. New York: Academic Press (1969).

Van Riper, C., Supervision of clinical practice. Asha, 7, 75–77 (1965).

Villarreal, J., Seminar on Guidelines for Supervision of Clinical Practicum. Washington, D.C.: American Speech and Hearing Association (1964).

Ward, L., and Webster, E., The training of clinical personnel: I. Issues in conceptualization. Asha, 7, 38–40 (1965a).

Ward, L., and Webster, E., The training of clinical personnel: II. A concept of clinical preparation. Asha, 7, 103–106 (1965b).

Being a practitioner, responsible for the welfare of another, introduces both challenge and conflict. In his new role the student clinician is directly engaged and tested within the occupational arena of a therapeutic encounter.

chapter 3
THE CLINICIAN AND THE THERAPEUTIC PROCESS

This chapter is written specifically for the student clinician in training. The first part attempts to capture, from the clinician's point of view, the essence of entering clinical practicum. Later portions trace clinician development and describe a process of clinician development and clinical effectiveness. Finally, systems of interaction analysis and research utilizing interactive methodologies are presented. Influence by the most important external agent, the clinical supervisor, is examined in the following chapter.

BECOMING A CLINICIAN

Very little analysis has been undertaken and little has been written concerning what happens to the student clinician psychologically during his clinical practicum experience. The clinician in training may be conceived of as being in a similar position to that of the astronomer, surrounded by stars deep within his clinical universe and continually trying to learn more about it. Little is known about the clinician's universe.

Less is known about the way the trainee acquires knowledge and develops behavior appropriate to the role of the speech clinician. This section focuses on the personal and emotional aspects of the problems encountered by the clinician in the process of clinical training.

In an effort to learn more about the process of becoming a clinician, this author conducted some personal research which involved informal interviews with approximately 30 undergraduate students. These students ranged from 1 year to 1 academic quarter away from entering their first clinical practicum experience. During each individual interview two open-ended questions were posed. First, the student was asked how he felt about entering clinical practicum, and second, he was asked to substantiate his feelings and tell why he felt the way he did. Students unanimously indicated feelings of anxiety or fear, which were said to stem from one of three major sources: the prospective supervisor, the client, or themselves. Student anxiety was foreseen concerning the inability to attain supervisory standards. Students expressed the burden of responsibility for the welfare of their future clients and the feeling that under the management of novice clinicians like themselves, harm could easily prevail. Often students voiced fear of being unable to put necessary classroom learning into practice.

To the extent that these results are stable and fairly representative of similar student populations, it seems that the process of becoming a clinician generates a number of different kinds of anxieties for the clinical trainee. Personal conversations with students confirm the existence of such anxieties long before their entrance into clinical practicum. Unlike the typical classroom situation, which is concerned with helping the individual student examine and scrutinize his thoughts and ideas, clinical training also involves a change in personality as well as a change in behavior. The individual is asked to think about himself in a totally new and different context. He must decide what is expected of him as a clinician, what personal objectives he is to realize, and how most effectively to obtain these objectives. Furthermore, he must develop ideas and plans about what he will do and be as a clinician. The reality shock of being a practitioner, responsible for the welfare of another, introduces both challenge and conflict. In his new role the student clinician is directly engaged and tested within the occupational arena of a therapeutic encounter. The demands of therapy test his ability to plan, manage, and execute control of his own as well as his client's behavior. He knows he has entered the "doing" context of our profession.

These multiple aspects frequently exceed the student clinician's capacity to cope and adapt. The gap between the requirements of therapy, the student's expectations of therapy, and his actual clinical performance all create stress. This stress is often compounded by distorted perceptions of client and supervisor both, which serve as additional sources of anxiety. The trainee soon comes to realize that in fact there are many therapeutic roads that lead to Rome, and as Van Riper (1975) points out, this situation undoubtedly poses further threat to the neophyte seeking unrealistically for one clear picture of what speech clinicians must be. Although supervisors take pride in seeing a bit of themselves in their clinicians, the wise supervisor instructs the clinician to be himself and thereby maximize his therapeutic effect. The clinician soon seeks for personal role definition. The development of consistent concepts of oneself, as clinician, becomes synthesized with personal factors into a unique personal and professional role identity. A true clinical self evolves.

Usually after a number of experiences, as the learner continues in supervised practicum, role behavior develops. Role learning requires behaving, feeling, and perceiving the clinical world in a manner similar to that of other individuals occupying such a position within that world. Appropriate attitudes, values, and behaviors are learned from more experienced members within the profession; hence, an ideology is shared. Van Riper (1965) acknowledges such catalytic role learning when he states that, "the basic clinical attitudes and competencies are learned more through identification and empathy than by precept" (p. 77).

Caple (1972) provides a vivid picture of the trainee's movement through the training experience. He describes the individual upon entering the system as moving in a fairly uniform pattern corresponding to his lowest energy level. As beginning movement occurs, contact is made with various stimuli and elements in the program. The pattern is one of low energy, little conflict, and harmony. As growth and development occur, the individual moves in less uniform patterns corresponding to higher energy levels, increased tension, greater conflict, and less harmony. When an individual moves in a manner consistent with the dynamics of the training program, tension is minimal and harmony prevails. When the individual moves through the system in a manner that is inconsistent with it, increased tension results, conflicts may arise, and harmony is disrupted.

The development of a professional identity means a psychologically complex and often profound process of conformity and personal change in the individual's intentions, perceptions, assumptions, and behavior (Mosher and Purpel, 1972). The impact of these changes has its most profound effect during the first clinical practicum experience. At this time the student must deal with client needs, supervisory demands, and his own personal experiences and expectations. The student clinician, by virtue of his title, is forced to play dual roles in which he must integrate both student and professional identities. Through contact with his environment and various role models, professionalism begins to develop.

CLINICAL COMPETENCE AND THE THERAPEUTIC PROCESS

What does the speech clinician in training need to know? What skills must be obtained? Who is the effective clinician? What is clinical competence? These are the critically important issues that plague the training and development of speech clinicians. The importance of effective clinical work has long been recognized within the field of speech pathology (Powers, 1956; Spriestersbach, 1965; Van Hattum, 1966; Mowrer, 1972). Authorities have attempted to communicate the essence of the therapeutic experience (Van Riper, 1966, 1975; McReynolds, 1970; Guildston and Guildston, 1972; Mowrer, 1974). A formidable body of important clinical methodologies currently exists for working with all communication disorders within our field. However, efforts to identify the essence of clinical effectiveness have been fruitless. The great variability among clinical methodologies, clinical settings, supervisors, clinicians, and clients has complicated the application of rigid controls for the research necessary to explore these crucial questions. Much of what is known about the clinical process and therapeutic effectiveness is in the realm of insight and intuition, culled from accumulated experience. Ingram and Stunden (1967) have likened the clinician to a skilled craftsman, who relies on techniques and procedures that are based on incomplete fragments of knowledge and traditionally have been passed on from master clinician to student clinician in an apprenticeship fashion.

Clinical competence traditionally has been viewed as a series of molar clinician characteristics, such as: shows appropriate level of clinical involvement, uses materials creatively, establishes rapport, and so on (MacLearie, 1958; Brown, 1967; Haller, 1967; Turton, 1973; Klevans and Volz, 1974). The division of these competency-based criteria into discrete areas such as diagnosis, treatment, and interpersonal and professional relations has been suggested by Diedrich (1969) and by Perkins et al. (1970) and has received statistical support by Schriberg et al. (1975). Results of an exploratory factor-analytic study of competency-based criteria within the parameter of therapeutic treatment alone (Oratio, 1976a) has indicated that two major behavioral dimensions are regarded by supervisors as critical to the process of therapeutic treatment: technical skill and interpersonal relationship dimensions (Table 1). Despite the critical importance of the problem, this study represents a singular attempt to identify, through *a posteriori* experimentation, competency-based criteria that can be used to evaluate clinical effectiveness.

Such a view of clinical competence, however, may have some inherent limitations at its very outset. Little is known about the relationship between molar clinician characteristics and the moment-to-moment progression of the therapeutic process. Although research suggests a high correlation between ratings of molar teacher performance and molecular teaching behaviors, based on content analysis (Fortune, 1969; Wallen, 1969), the relationship between ratings of molar clinician performance and discrete therapeutic interaction in speech pathology has yet to be determined. Futhermore, it has been shown that the clinician's academic status significantly influences the supervisory evaluation of therapeutic effectiveness, irrespective of the clinician's therapeutic behavior (Oratio, 1976b). This finding indicates that a significant portion of supervisors' evaluation of molar clinician characteristics is predetermined based on training level alone. Finally, validity of criteria is a vexing issue. Research must be undertaken to obtain the predictive potential of molar competency-based criteria. It remains to be determined whether clinician performance criteria can be validated through measures of client improvement. Perhaps an ultimate research strategy into clinical competence involves first determining

Table 1. Factor structure of interpersonal and technical skill variables (From Oratio, 1967a; reprinted with permission)

Factors	Variables
I. Technical skill	1. Uses every opportunity to obtain target responses from the client
	2. Modifies planned strategy to maximize target responses
	3. Uses materials creatively to stimulate client interest
	4. Changes therapeutic procedure to meet client needs
	5. Resolves unexpected problems in therapy
	6. Applies theoretical knowledge of the disorder to therapeutic practice
	7. Appropriately reinforces the client's approximations to the target response
	8. Uses effective schedule of reinforcement
	9. Accomplishes the session's goals
	10. Implements carryover procedures in therapy
II. Interpersonal relationship	11. Establishes rapport as evidenced verbally and nonverbally
	12. Shows respect for the client as evidenced verbally and nonverbally
	13. Uses appropriate speech characteristics: rate, pitch, volume, and so on
	14. Communicates at the client's cognitive and linguistic levels
	15. Shows emotional stability during therapy
	16. Maintains appropriate personal appearance
	17. Shows appropriate attitudes in therapy: enthusiasm, positive outlook, and so on
	18. Shows appropriate level of clinical involvement

parameters of significant therapeutic behavior on a molar level, and then content-analyzing the more discrete molecular components for clinical training purposes.

In dealing with the issue of clinical effectiveness, effectiveness cannot be separated from methodology, pathology, goals, or select clinician and client characteristics. From the field of counseling, Krumboltz (1966) writes:

> What we need to know is which procedures and techniques, when used to accomplish which kinds of behavior change, are most effective with what kind of client when applied by what kind of counselor (p. 5).

In addressing this problem from the viewpoint of psychotherapy, Strupp and Bergin (1969) similarly indicate that, "the problem of psychotherapy research . . . should be reformulated as, what specific interventions produce specific changes in specific patients under specific conditions?" Finally, Paul (1967) suggests that all outcome research be directed toward, "what treatment, by whom, is most effective for this individual with that specific problem and under which set of circumstances?" (p. 111). Perhaps we, too, must address ourselves to a somewhat more sophisticated question in the same manner that these workers have. Somehow the research endeavor becomes more meaningful when we ask, "What are the effective therapeutic characteristics, applied by a particular clinician, in order to achieve a particular goal with a particular client at a particular point in therapy?"

SPEECH THERAPY AS A TRANSACTIVE PROCESS

Speech therapy has been defined as a transactive process containing interpersonal and technical elements. It can be further defined as the actual therapeutic performance and its results. It consists both of what clinicians do and what clients do, observably and in interaction. Additionally, it consists of numerous internal variables. The dual track nature of the supervisory-therapeutic paradigm presented earlier indicates that interactions are of both an internal (feeling, emotional) and external (verbal, gestural) nature. Such interactions between clinicians and clients are not random but show recurring and characteristic patterns (Boone and Goldberg, 1969; Boone and Stech, 1970; Schubert, Miner, and Till, 1973; Grandstaff, 1974). For example, the clinician may stimulate the client with an antecedent such as modeling and the client may respond on target, wherein the clinician then asks for the client's self-evaluation of the production and follows with a confirming reinforcer. Whatever the clinician or client characteristics and content or context variables, therapeutic performance reflects some such pattern of behaviors and their effect. It seems likely that immediate therapeutic effect (the learning of and ability to incorporate and maintain a new speech pattern) largely results from both internal and external interactions during the therapeutic process, that is, what the clinician does, says, thinks, and feels, and what the client does, says, thinks, and feels. An important part of what determines the effect or outcome of therapy may be either explicit or implicit in these transactions. These events, which constitute the action of therapy, can be captured, categorized, quantified, analyzed, and preserved for later study through the application of transactional models and self-confrontation procedures.

WHAT THE CLINICIAN NEEDS TO KNOW

Although what clinicians and clients say and do during therapy is the most immediate and valid index of both progress and performance, such narrow analysis accounts for only part of the therapeutic procedure and its effect. How clinicians and clients interact (the internal or interpersonal variables that are generated) is as much a matter of concern as what they interact about. Factor-analytic research, previously cited, has uncovered two distinct dimensions that contribute to therapeutic effectiveness; one of these is the interpersonal dimension, the other concerns technical skills. These dimensions are both an integral part of the therapeutic process.

Across pathologies, diverse therapeutic approaches have been known to meet with success. A common element in these approaches concerns the interpersonal relationship established between clinician and client and the interactions, such as warmth and confidence, that are generated. Only in those few attempts to apply modern automated technology to speech therapy (Holland and Matthews, 1963; Stunden, 1966) does this situation fail to hold true. Even in the supposed strictly behavioristic approaches, interpersonal variables cannot be excluded from the therapeutic intervention. In this context Allport (1962) writes: "The trouble with our current theories of learning is not so much that they are wrong, but that they are partial" (p. 380). The essential point is that regardless of therapeutic persuasion, internal and external interactions comprise the clinician's approach, and the clinician is always a significant member of the therapeutic dyad.

Some researchers and practitioners have hypothesized that the quality of the internal or interpersonal interaction is the most potent source of therapeutic effect and is most determinative of the therapeutic outcome. From the field of counseling, Truax (1970) writes:

> As the evidence accumulates, it becomes clear that the counselor's interpersonal skill in relating to clients has much to do with inducing positive client change. While specialized techniques and expert knowledge are believed important, it is already clear that they are secondary (p. 6).

From the field of speech pathology, Ward and Webster (1965) indicate that clinical effectiveness depends first on the clinician's ability to create and maintain a satisfying interpersonal relationship, and second on the ability to apply knowledge of the nature and treatment of speech and hearing disorders to the client. Patterson (1973), in discussing the therapeutic relationship, states it as follows:

> Such a relationship may be characterized not so much by what techniques the therapist uses, as by what he is, not so much by what he does as by the way he does it (p. 536).

This is not to say that an optimal interpersonal relationship is both necessary and sufficient for the remediation of speech defects. Information and instruction are vital for effecting a change in the client's speech pattern. Although techniques may serve to direct a change in speech behavior along the lines which the therapist desires, it is the therapeutic relationship that makes change and influence possible. This concept has particular significance for the carryover stages of therapy, when the clinician releases control and minimizes overt gestural cues. The responsibility is then placed on the client, where interactions are largely subtle and judgments internal.

It should be pointed out that assumptions that the clinician is the presumed "cause" of what happens in therapy are erroneous. There is simply a relationship between what the clinician is, feels, and does, how he conveys this to the client, and the effectiveness of the client's therapy. More importantly, there are a multitude of internal, intervening variables that preclude a strictly behavioral analysis of the therapeutic process. Research has not yet been .able to uncover all of these multivariate factors, their interaction, effect, and how they can be used to predict and control the therapeutic outcome. The effective variables of speech therapy are multiple and complex in their interaction. In the absence of this total array, however, there do seem to be some variables that can be isolated and presumed to account for at least some of the variance in therapeutic effectiveness. Additionally, there is a growing body of evidence that substantiates the importance of the interpersonal relationship in therapeutic learning.

INTERPERSONAL ATTRACTION

One of the most stable findings in all of social and behavioral science research involves the positive relationship between similarity and attraction. People like each other in direct proportion to their similarity on a particular attribute (Byrne, 1965). Conversely, the more similar people are to one another, the greater will be their level of attraction. This research yields well defined and consistent results. The relationship cited is almost a straight line linear function capable of formulation in descriptive equations.

Additional findings have shown that the more people are attracted to one another, the more they communicate and the greater is their influence upon one another during interpersonal communication (Berscheid and Walster, 1969; McCroskey, Larson and Knapp, 1971; Rogers and Shoemaker, 1971). These findings have been applied to a number of therapeutic situations and there is evidence to suggest that therapy-like learning is enhanced by positive interpersonal relationships, and that the quality of the interpersonal relationship is related to client performance (Sapolsky, 1960; Lott and Lott, 1966; Lott, 1969; Mendelsohn and Rankin, 1969). Interpersonal attraction has been shown to be a multidimensional construct involving three basic dimensions: a social or personal liking dimension; a physical dimension based on dress and physical features; and a task-orientation dimension related to how easy or worthwhile working with someone would be (McCroskey and McCaine, 1974). These interpersonal dimensions should be foremost in the clinician's mind while working with the client. He should actively scrutinize the level of interpersonal attraction between himself and his client and attempt to gain some assessment of the client's perceptions.

THE EFFECTIVE CLINICIAN

The effective clinician is, first, one who responds appropriately to multiple client factors within the clinical setting. These include overt factors such as the individual client's behavior, attention, speech pattern, and so on, as well as internal factors such as the client's attitudes, emotions, motivations, anxieties, likes, and dislikes. Second, since the clinician's behavior is of both an internal and external nature (that is, it involves feelings and emotions as well as overt verbal and gestural responses), he must seek to control and blend the interaction of his behavior with the client's behavior. Erickson and Van Riper (1967) described the control of interaction as follows:

> The interpersonal processes of speech therapy require empathy, moment-by-moment choices of techniques, continual judgments, and many other subtle interactions which are exceedingly difficult to reconstruct and depict outside of the therapy room (p. 33).

It is the clinician who takes responsibility for controlling client interaction. Research in the fields of counseling and education has shown that, within an interpersonal dyad, it is the person in the superior position who determines the level of functioning of the second person (Truax and Carkhuff, 1965; Blumberg, 1974).

In attempting to give further insight into the interactive complexities of therapy, some theorists have indicated that the clinician must simultaneously heed both the patient and himself (Harrison and Carek, 1966). Others have suggested that the clinician must have a three-point view of the encounter, in which he can perceive it as an observer looking in on the therapeutic dyad, perceive his own behavior from the client's point of view, as well as perceive the therapeutic situation from his own viewpoint. Whether it is possible to achieve these perspectives is unknown. The important point is that the quality of interaction gives rise to a particular climate which may have positive or negative effects.

THERAPEUTIC ENVIRONMENT

Clinician-client interactions are conceived of as dynamic and in constant motion. Their movement is capable of generating novel therapeutic ideas, judgments, and strategies. Interactions generated by each member of the therapeutic dyad give rise to a particular psychological, therapeutic climate. Therapeutic efficiency is reached when these clinician-client multivariate interactions are held in harmony and balance by a common purpose, thereby creating a state of equilibrium. Figure 3 illustrates this situation. Here we see that when the clinician conveys positive affect and uses appropriate techniques, and when the client responds appropriately to these circumstances, a positive therapeutic climate prevails. In this illustration, it is conceptualized that interactions are appropriately selected, efficiently utilized, focused, and held in harmony by a common purpose, the therapeutic goal.

Figure 4 illustrates a different therapeutic environment.

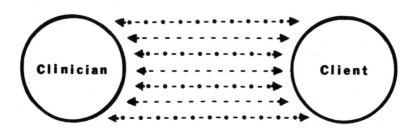

Figure 3. Clinician-client interactions illustrating a positive therapeutic environment.

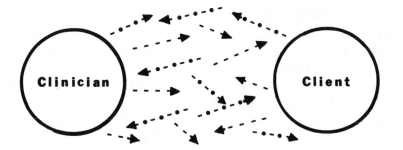

Figure 4. Clinician-client interactions illustrating a negative therapeutic environment.

When specific clinician-client variables are out of balance, a negative therapeutic climate is created. Here we see inefficient, random interactions between clinician and client, characterized by a lack of interactive focus. This situation is not unlike that of random socialization, in which little therapeutic effect is evidenced.

CLINICIAN INTERACTIVE VARIABLES

What then are the multivariate clinician-client factors that are capable of either a random or harmonious interaction and that seem to account for the initiation and occurrence of the therapeutic process and environment? Although no single theory can encompass all of the details of human interaction, perhaps the essential ingredients of effective therapeutic intervention can be specified by a relatively small class of variables.

There is currently a clear-cut and striking body of evidence which indicates that certain core facilitative conditions have implications for all interpersonal learning processes, including teacher-student, parent-child, supervisor-clinician, or clinician-client relationships (Carkhuff and Truax, 1966; Carkhuff, 1969a, 1969b, 1971). What is most striking in the research findings to date is that this core of interpersonal skills is motivating, therapeutic, or change-inducing, no matter what area—psychotic behavior, friendship relationships, or arithmetic and reading achievement—is being measured (Carkhuff and Berenson, 1967; Truax and Carkhuff, 1967; Truax and Mitchell, 1970). These first four dimensions then appear to be active and effective ingredients in all human learning processes. As clinician variables, they encompass the interpersonal dimension uncovered by factor-analytic research (Oratio, 1976a) and are actively conveyed and generated to the client in communications during the therapeutic encounter. Instruments for assessing gross facilitative functioning within these four dimensions are available for both the supervisor's and clinician's use (Carkhuff and Berenson, 1967; Carkhuff, 1969a, 1969b).

Empathic Understanding

Empathic understanding involves the clinician's ability to identify with the client. It is the ability to experience the client's difficulty in the same way that the client experiences it. It is an intimate sensitivity to the needs of the client and an understanding of how it feels to be the client.

Positive Regard

Positive regard involves an acceptance of and a respect for the client as a person and an individual in spite of his behavior and difficulties. Coupled with this is a concern for and interest in the client as an individual and a desire to help influence and change him.

Genuineness

Genuineness refers to the clinician's ability to be freely and deeply himself in his relationship with the client: to be open to experience and spontaneous in his relationship; to be authentic, sincere, and honest; and to be willing to share himself with the client.

Concreteness

Concreteness concerns the clinician's ability to lead the client to the target goal which is appropriate at that particular point in therapy. Such concrete behavior not only leads but enables the client to achieve the goal.

Technical Skill

Technical skill involves the clinician's knowledge of the nature of the client's speech disorder. It includes knowledge and utilization of methods, approaches, and techniques that are based on research and experience and can be used to change speech behavior and ultimately remediate the client's speech disorder. The factor-analytic research previously discussed (Oratio, 1976a) indicated that a core of 10 technical skills (see Table 1) was perceived by over 150 supervisors as critically determinative of therapeutic effectiveness. These technical skills have implications for both the execution and measurement of therapeutic behavior. It is essential that the clinician have an integrated storehouse of such methods and principles that can be immediately called upon and used in the remediation of the variety of speech and language disorders encountered. Such cognitive flexibility, involving the ability to adapt and utilize principles and methodologies to the reaction of the client, has been thought to be a significant factor in various learning environments (Sprinthall, Whiteley, and Mosher, 1966).

Confidence

Confidence concerns the clinician's belief that the client's speech behavior will change and that his therapy will be effective in producing that change. Emerick has referred to this condition as "focused optimism" (Emerick and Hood, 1974). This belief and expectation of client change is manifested in the clinician's level of confidence in the principles and methods he employs.

In summary, an empathic understanding of the client's problem, a respect for the client as an individual, the clinician's ability to share himself with the client and lead the client to achieving the therapeutic goal, have been shown to be core facilitatory dimensions in a variety of interpersonal learning contexts. In addition, it is proposed that the clinician's knowledge of technical skills, his ability to adapt therapeutic principles to the reaction of the client, as well as the level of confidence he conveys in his approach, are critical to therapeutic effectiveness. These six variables are present in varying degrees within the ongoing interaction between clinician and client.

CLIENT VARIABLES

Three specific client variables are also present in varying degrees within the therapeutic encounter. It is speculated that these variables affect clinician behavior and enhance or retard the therapeutic process.

Perception

The client's perception of the clinician is most crucial in the clinician's impact upon the client. It is actually not clinician behavior but ultimately the client's perception of the clinician as a competent, caring professional that will determine client change. The client must feel the clinician's competence and concern in wanting to help him. Since it is the client who changes his own behavior, his attitudes and perceptions are of primary importance.

Belief in Change

The client must believe that a change in his speech behavior is possible. His belief is somewhat related to his perception of the clinician's level of confidence and the clinician's belief that he can change the client's speech behavior. It is the client's faith in the fact that he will and can improve. Often we feel the consequences of children in our clinics who convey the negative belief, "I can't do it!"

Participation

Finally, the client must be willing to participate and be an active member in the therapeutic process. In order for change to occur, the client must participate intellectually, emotionally, verbally, and motorically. He must be willing to either examine and correct old behavior, or explore, experiment, and develop new behaviors.

To understand the effectiveness of speech therapy, we must look at numerous clinician-client variables. Effective therapy depends upon the interaction of a number of variables whose optimal mix varies in each situation. It has been suggested that when the clinician can create and maintain an interactive equilibrium between his own and the client's interactions, a positive therapeutic environment is created and therapeutic interaction takes place. In order for this therapeutic interaction to occur, the clinician must function at high levels of empathy, positive regard, genuineness, and concreteness, must demonstrate a knowledge of technical skills, and must exude confidence in his approach. Likewise, the client must perceive the clinician's competence, confidence, and high level of functioning. He must have a belief in the fact that his speech can be changed, and he must show a high level of participatition in helping to change his speech behavior. In support of this notion, research in social ecology depicts man in interaction with his environment, giving rise to a particular kind of environment which functions to facilitate or retard treatment effects (Wolfe, 1966; Mischel, 1968; Moos, 1969, 1973, 1974). Furthermore, studies in interpersonal attraction indicate that variables within the interpersonal dimension contribute powerfully to therapeutic learning.

PROCESS OF CLINICIAN DEVELOPMENT

The most important issue of clinical supervision involves the process by which the clinician effectively develops, and how both the supervisor and supervisory procedures function to enhance this developmental process. Clinician development is viewed as an ongoing process which has its initiation during the period of clinical practicum and proceeds throughout the clinician's entire professional career. During this time the clinician should focus on clinical development within three major skill areas. The process of clinical development in its early stages involves the integration of technical knowledge and clinical skill through the clinician's self-exploration. Each of these areas is identified as follows.

Technical Knowledge

The effective clinician needs to have an understanding of theories, methodologies, principles, and techniques that are applicable to his particular client. He needs to understand the nature of the therapeutic relationship and the core facilitatory dimensions, previously mentioned, which are active within this relationship.

Clinical Skill

Not only must the clinician have a knowledge and understanding of the clinician dimensions previously mentioned, but through continued practice he must develop skill in their use. Through such practice he must be capable of making the moment-to-moment decisions that are a part of the therapeutic encounter. He must be skilled not only in the observation of the client's speech behavior but also in the observation of the client's perceptions, beliefs, and level of participation. The observation of these behaviors provides the foundation for clinical decision making.

Self-Exploration

The clinician must seek to understand himself, both his cognitive and conative aspects. He must have a grasp of his own needs, drives, and motivations as well as an understanding of his level of technical knowledge. Finally, he must explore all of these aspects of self and seek to integrate them into a unique clinical self.

It is necessary to add a fourth dimension to these three ingredients, the supervisory dimension. Both the supervisor and the supervisory procedures play a major role in the clinician's development within the above areas. The supervisor and the procedures he utilizes should focus on facilitating the clinician's integrative processes.

In addition, the supervisor should maintain an awareness of the level of clinician development in each of the above areas, and he should structure supervisory procedures to meet the clinician's needs. Perhaps a formula may best serve to illustrate and summarize the process of clinician growth and development. It is hypothesized that:

$$CD = \frac{\dfrac{(P + Tk + Cs)}{Se} \times \dfrac{(SP)}{Si}}{T}$$

Where:

CD = clinician development
P = clinician personality
Tk = clinician technical knowledge
Cs = clinical skill
Se = clinician self-exploration
SP = supervisory procedures
Si = supervisor influence
T = time

These seem to be the factors that influence the clinician's development. Such development occurs when the clinician's personality, technical knowledge, and clinical practice become integrated through self-exploration. The supervisory procedures and the supervisor's personal influence are conceived of as having a significant impact on clinician development; they may serve to facilitate or retard the integrative process of clinical development. These dynamics all take place over time.

The supervisory element is a most important element within the process of clinical development. It is particularly important to students who are engaged in clinical practicum and are therefore beginners in the process. It decreases in importance as self-exploration, growth, and responsible decision making take place. Supervision must be structured to develop the process of self-supervision within the clinician by facilitating the clinician's level of self-exploration. This process of self-scrutiny results in a movement away from supervisory dependence and a movement toward professional autonomy-independence. As the clinician approaches maturity, supervision assumes less importance, becomes less intense, and eventually is discontinued. The elements of technical knowledge and clinical skill then become more highly integrated with the clinician's personality and further refined through the process of self-exploration. These elements are conceptualized as seeking further and further integration and refinement throughout the clinician's professional career. Thus even the seasoned clinician remains in the process of becoming.

The clinician who can perform the exploratory function independent of supervision, whose behavior can be captured by the first half of the equation, has become clinically mature. Clinician self-study is considered a crucial goal of an effective supervisory experience. The implication is that the supervisor must initiate application of the principles of self-scrutiny; this then enables the clinician to eventually apply such principles to himself. The clinician's self-study and integration of his attitudes, emotions, behavior, and knowledge are crucial to the development of his clinical identity. Can supervision facilitate such integration?

Chapter 4 explores this important issue. Before examining supervisor-clinician dynamics, however, the range of interactive methodologies that have been developed and utilized as both clinician and supervisory tools are first presented with current research on interaction analysis. These descriptive instruments are currently our most useful means of quantifying and analyzing communications within the therapeutic environment. It is therefore necessary that the clinician incorporate one of these instruments into his own clinical armamentarium.

OVERVIEW OF INTERACTION ANALYSIS

Interaction analysis is concerned with quantifying and analyzing transitory communications contained within a variety of interpersonal learning contexts. The bulk of interactive theory has come from the field of education, where category systems have been developed for quantifying both verbal and nonverbal transactions. There are currently over 80 interaction systems available (Simon and Boyer, 1967) for quantifying and analyzing communications contained within classroom teaching, psychotherapy, and speech pathology settings. These systems vary in the number of observational categories employed, but they typically use a two-by-two matrix for summarizing and analyzing transactive data.

Interaction analysis can be traced to the field of education, where H. H. Anderson (1939, 1945, 1946a, 1946b) studied the dominative and integrative behavior of teachers. Withall (1951) refined Anderson's observational system into a seven-category system called the Social-Emotional Climate Index, which contained learner-centered and teacher-centered dimensions. Flanders (1965) further refined both of these systems and developed the Flanders Interaction Analysis Category System. This 10-category system contains means for quantifying both indirect and direct teacher behavior as well as student behavior. More recently, Blumberg (1970) developed a 15-category system which has its origin in Flanders' (1965) two-dimensional conceptualization of indirect and direct interaction. This system has been used to analyze both supervisor-teacher and teacher-student communication. Both the Flanders and Blumberg systems have enjoyed great popularity and have been used in the fields of education as well as in speech pathology.

INTERACTION ANALYSIS
IN SPEECH PATHOLOGY

Since the advent of early interactive systems, there has been a feverish interest in applying interactive methodologies to helping professions such as psychology, psychiatry, counseling, and speech pathology. Of particular interest has been the use of videotape feedback in conjunction with pattern analysis for purposes of observing and changing clinical behavior as well as for developing clinical skills (Diedrich, 1969). These procedures have been widely referred to as videotaped self-confrontation. Numerous transactional models have been developed in speech pathology that permit abstraction of the enormously complex array of fleeting events which take place in therapy.

One of the first transactional models was designed by Johnson (1969), who utilized a 40-category multidimensional scoring system for observing the clinical process in speech pathology. This system employs both verbal (stimulus, response, consequation) and nonverbal events as a means of codifying clinical transactions. The multitude of categories within the system allows for detailed data analysis. Intra-judge reliability scores were reported to be .84 and above; however, inter-judge reliability scores were found to be low and were attributed to differences in supervisory philosophies for scoring clinical events.

Between the years 1969 and 1971, a series of studies were conducted on a 10-category system which has been referred to as the Boone-Prescott Interaction Analysis System (Boone and Prescott, 1971, 1972). This system has enjoyed much popularity within speech pathology and can be used to analyze both individual and group therapy. It employs five categories that are related to clinician behavior and five categories that are related to client behavior. Reliability of the instrument has been shown to be high. A 5-minute segment of therapy yields data that are representative of the entire therapy session. This simple system has undergone a number of adaptations. Prescott (1970) expanded the 10 categories to 19, while retaining high intra- and inter-judge reliability of .94 and .96, respectively. Prescott and Tesauro (1974) reduced and modified this 19-category system to a 17-category system, which can be used reliably to describe and quantify the events of clinician-parent-child interaction during aural rehabilitation.

Shortly after the Boone-Prescott system was developed, Schubert, Miner, and Till (1973) developed the Analysis of

Behavior of Clinicians (ABC) System which consists of 12 categories. Eight categories in this system pertain to clinician behavior, three categories pertain to client behavior, and the final category is reserved for the scoring of silence. The unique feature in this system is that it contains a temporal element. Interactive data are recorded in a time-based fashion at 3-second intervals. Each number corresponds to the inter-action which occurs during the 3-second interval immediately preceeding the recording. Schubert and Laird (1975) have recently reported that using the ABC System a 3-minute segment of therapy is representative of the entire therapy session during articulation and language therapy.

Lingwall and Engmann (1971) have developed a reliable operant model which categorizes three classes of clinician events: antecedent events, response events, and subsequent events. They suggest that this system can be used for re-search, training, or clinical treatment purposes. For research, the system can be used to specify clinical events descrip-tively; in training, to quantify changes in clinician behavior; and in treatment, to specify a variety of client responses.

Mulhern (1972) utilized a modified form of Medley's Observation Schedule and Record 4V (OScaR) called the Therapy Oscar (ToScaR), (Medley and Mitzel, 1963). Using this modification, Mulhern quantified clinician reinforcement patterns as a function of client verbalization during group language therapy. This system was found to be effective and has implications for examining interaction during group therapy.

Grandstaff (1974) developed an analysis model that con-sists of 11 categories, nine of which pertain to clinician behavior and two which quantify total client responses and correct versus incorrect client response ratios. Although this model is operantly based, four categories deal with clinician decision making (that is, increases or decreases task diffi-culty, indicates why a particular response was appropriate, and so on). This system has been shown to be effective in discerning and discriminating clinical behaviors among various groups of clinicians.

In addition to the above systems, the Flander's Interaction Analysis System has been used effectively to analyze stuttering therapy (Giandomenico, 1970). In 1974, Kaplan and Dreyer developed a multidimensional system which is an adaptation of a number of already existing systems. In their research, which has been previously discussed (Chapter 2), this multidimensional system was used to analyze both verbal and nonverbal behavior.

Each of the above systems employs a different number of categories (ranging as high as 40). They each quantify different types of behavioral events and utilize a slightly different means of scoring. All of them can be used for purposes of observation and analysis, and all yield valuable data for helping speech clinicians in training to modify their own as well as their client's behavior.

With the multitude of interactive systems available, it is surprising that little comparative research has been conducted on these systems. One unique attempt to compare interaction systems is available in the literature. Schubert and Glick (1973) compared the information obtained from the ABC and the Boone-Prescott Systems. These two systems differ in the number of categories they employ (although eight of the categories are similar) and in the method employed for scoring. Since the ABC System contains a time-based scoring factor, it was not known whether both systems would yield similar information. Videotape recordings were made of eight student clinicians involved in articulation and language therapy with 4- to 6-year-old children. It was found that the two systems yielded approximately the same information when the therapy was based on stimulus-response-reinforcement, with a minimum of irrelevant behavior. The ABC System gave more information when the session was poorly planned and executed. Both systems were found to provide objective information useful in changing clinical behavior.

EFFECTS OF INTERACTION
ANALYSIS ON CLINICIAN BEHAVIOR

Three studies have been conducted to determine the combined effects of the Boone-Prescott Interaction Analysis System and videotaped/audiotaped self-confrontation feedback methods on the training of speech clinicians (Boone and Goldberg, 1969; Boone and Stech, 1970; Boone and Prescott, 1971). Results of these studies indicated that:

1. There was no significant difference in basic change measures between the clinicians using videotape and those using audiotape in self-confrontation procedures.
2. There were significant increases in the clinician's knowledge of learning theory.
3. The clinicians were able to change from using positive reinforcement and punishment schedules 100 percent and 0 percent, respectively, to using both forms of responses at about a 50 percent ratio.
4. The use of a category system tends to keep clinicians "reality oriented" in terms of actual and ideal performance and allows clinicians to evaluate and change their own behavior.

Giandomenico (1970) trained 13 speech clinicians in the Flanders' Interaction Analysis Category System and investigated the effects of this training on the clinicians' verbal behavior during stuttering therapy. The relationship between the clinicians' concept of "ideal" and "actual" verbal behavior for both control and experimental groups, before and after training was examined. Clinicians in the experimental group received training in the Flanders' System, and those in the control group did not. Findings indicated:

1. No significant relationship was found, for either group, between "ideal" and "actual" verbal behavior prior to training.

2. After training, clinicians in the experimental group showed significant changes in moving closer to their "ideal" verbal behavior.

3. A significant change occurred in the control group's "actual" verbal behavior. Every clinician in the group became more direct in their responses over time.

In addition to these studies in speech pathology, a review of self-confrontation procedures in the fields of education and psychology generally supports its use as an effective means of changing behavior (Fuller and Manning, 1970; Kagan, 1970; Marshall and Hegrenes, 1970; Soloman and MacDonald, 1970; Leonard, Gies, and Paden, 1971; Young and Young, 1971; Fuller et al., 1973).

BEHAVIORAL DIFFERENCES BETWEEN EXPERIENCED AND INEXPERIENCED CLINICIANS

Over a short period of time, a number of researchers have used interaction systems to investigate differences in the clinical behaviors of experienced and inexperienced clinicians. Using the Prescott Nineteen Category System, Olsen (1972) studied behavioral differences between experienced (above 275 clinical clock hours) and inexperienced (below 275 clinical clock hours) clinicians engaged in therapy with clients having articulation, delayed language, prosody, and voice disorders. Second, he investigated whether randomly selected 5- and 10-minute segments of therapy were representative of entire therapy sessions. Findings indicated that the Prescott System was capable of differentiating differences in interactions and sequences of interactions between experienced and inexperienced clinicians. The correlations of 5- and 10-minute segments of therapy with the entire therapy sessions were found to be sufficiently high to consider a 5-minute segment to be a representation of the entire therapy session.

Schubert, Miner, and Prather (1972) measured behavioral differences between 20 undergraduate clinicians (10 beginning and 10 advanced) using the ABC System. Comparisons were made of interactions during beginning and intermediate 5-minute segments of therapy. No significant differences were found between initial and intermediate 5-minute segments; however, clinicians were observed to be instructing and demonstrating more frequently at the beginning of the sessions and using more authority as they were further into the session. Significant differences were found between beginning and advanced clinicians in 10 of the 12 categories of the ABC System (instruction, reinforcement, and so on). Beginning clinicians were also observed to modify their lesson significantly less often than advanced clinicians.

In an earlier investigation, Stech (1969) studied behavioral changes in the therapeutic performance of student clinicians under videotaped self-confrontation. He hypothesized that changes in clinician behavior are related to three factors: 1) academic achievement and aptitude, 2) emotional control, and 3) total course work and clinical practicum hours. Results indicated a high correlation between independent and dependent variables. Initial reinforcement ratios were found to be related to personality and experience variables, with high reinforcement rates being exhibited by extraverted, highly self-esteemed, and highly experienced subjects. Changes involving the use of more negative reinforcement were found to be related to increased training. Changes in the use of less positive reinforcement were found to be inversely related to intelligence and personality variables but positively related to clinical experience.

Grandstaff (1974) investigated differences in therapeutic behavior between three groups of clinicians with different levels of training and experience: 10 untrained student clinicians with 2 to 10 clock hours of clinical practicum, 10 moderately trained student clinicians with 75 to 100 clock

hours of practicum, and 10 trained clinicians who were
university graduates, state certified, and had 2 years of employment in the public schools. A 1-hour sample of each
subject engaged in articulation therapy was tape recorded and
analyzed by three judges according to Grandstaff's interaction model. Results indicated that:

1. Trained clinicians evoked a significantly higher number
    of correct responses than moderately trained clinicians.
2. Moderately trained clinicians evoked a significantly
    higher number of correct responses than untrained
    clinicians.
3. Untrained clinicians spoke a significantly higher
    number of words that were unrelated to changing
    speech behavior than did the moderately trained or
    trained speech clinicians.
4. In general, the more experienced clinicians gave more
    feedback to the client concerning the degree to which
    he was approximating the target response and more
    feedback concerning why the error had occurred.

Mercer and Schubert (1974) investigated the frequency
and type of nonverbal behaviors of graduate and undergraduate clinicians engaged in therapy. It was hypothesized
that the clinicians rated highest by supervisors on 10 clinical
competencies (establishes rapport, uses appropriate techniques, accomplishes goals, and so on) would differ in their
frequency and use of nonverbal behaviors from clinicians
rated lowest. Nonverbal behaviors included responses such as
smiles, positive head nod, negative nod, eye contact, postural
change, forward lean, positive touch, negative touch, and so
on. A total of 14 student clinicians, eight ranked high
(mostly graduate students) and six ranked low, served as
subjects for the study. Each subject was videotaped while
assigned to therapy with a client of preschool or school age.
Reliability scores were high for the preselected nonverbal

behaviors. Mercer and Schubert drew the following conclusions from the analysis of the data:

1. High rated and low rated clinicians differ in the number of nonverbal behaviors they use.
2. High rated clinicians use significantly more of the nonverbal behaviors which serve as social reinforcers and which serve to signal social interaction, such as smiles, positive head nods, and eye contact.
3. Predictions can be made as to whether a clinician is high or low rated based on the number of particular nonverbal behaviors he employs.
4. The ratings of clinicians by supervisors may be influenced by the clinician's use or lack of use of nonverbal behaviors.

Davis (1968) investigated the judgments made of clinician-client interactions by two panels of experienced speech and hearing clinicians. Sixty audiotaped samples of therapy were collected from different clinical settings geographically far apart. Samples were separated according to experienced and inexperienced therapists. Fifty of the samples were speech and hearing therapy, the other 10 were not. The judges were required to evaluate the samples on five questions concerning: 1) organization of the therapy, 2) quality of the therapy, 3) adequacy of the amount of the clinicians' talk, 4) appropriateness of the clinicians' interactions, and 5) degree of rapport. Two other questions required identification of speech and hearing therapy from those samples which were not, and discrimination of the clinician from the client. Results indicated that: 1) the questions elicited significantly different but highly correlated ratings, 2) reliability of ratings by the judges was low, 3) mean ratings of quality for experienced clinicians were significantly higher than for less experienced clinicians, 4) mean ratings for rapport were highest, and 5) the panels were able to identify speech and hearing therapy from other therapies and were able to discriminate the client from the clinician.

These studies indicate that regardless of how one defines experienced or inexperienced clinicians, or whether verbal or nonverbal interactions are measured, more highly trained clinicians are perceived both by supervisors and clinicians as behaving more consistently with the goals of speech therapy than inexperienced clinicians do. Observed differences have been shown to exist for the amount and type of reinforcement used, the amount of socialization and correct responses which occurred during therapy, the amount of feedback given to the client, the modification of therapy to meet the client's needs, and generally the overall quality of therapy delivered to the client. In most cases these discrete behaviors are based on a single scattered finding and therefore require replication. These studies, however, do corroborate the findings of our own extensive research (Oratio and Hood, in press) in which 152 supervisors evaluated the therapeutic performance of 207 speech clinicians. Regression analysis indicated that supervisors perceived three behaviors as contributing most significantly to the clinicians' accomplishment of the therapeutic goal: an effective schedule of reinforcement, implementation of carryover procedures in therapy, and modification of the therapeutic procedure in order to meet the client's needs.

The above studies, taken as a group, demonstrate that some aspect or aspects of training result in achieving higher levels of professional, clinical behavior. As clinicians move through the training program, their clinical behaviors are observed to improve. The stable constants which emerge from these data show that modification of the therapeutic procedure to meet the client's needs, and reinforcement are critical therapeutic behaviors. Second, behaviors of experienced clinicians differ from the clinical behaviors of inexperienced clinicians.

CONCLUSIONS

Research in clinical work as well as in supervision suggests that interaction analysis be the focus of these human transactive processes. Research findings lend support to the use of interaction analysis and self-confrontation as effective tools for training and supervising speech clinicians. The major problem confronting interaction analysis as an approach is that the significant categories and basic rules for analysis and summation of verbal interaction between clinicians and clients are still unknown. Unfortunately, our theories of clinical effectiveness are currently inadequate, and criteria for measuring effectiveness remain imprecise. The construct of *clinical competence* seems to defy objective measure. No statements have deeper implications for clinical supervision. Anderson (1974) has indicated that the lack of established clinical competencies complicates the supervisory function. Only after we achieve a greater understanding of therapeutic processes and their effects on remediation will we be in a much better position to enhance clinical supervision and clinical effectiveness.

The present review of the research indicates that interactive systems have been used for descriptive analyses of clinician behavior at discrete levels of training and as interactive tools to measure the effectiveness of specific training procedures, such as self-confrontation or micro-training. Further descriptive analyses should be undertaken at this time in order to investigate, for example, the effects of doubling interaction patterns, the effects of longer or shorter interaction patterns on client performance, the effects of a wide variety of patterns as opposed to few patterns, and an examination of those interaction patterns that emerge from successful and unsuccessful therapy sessions. In all cases, computer programs (Weller, 1969; Olsen, 1972; Campbell, 1975) can be used to accomplish such extensive analyses.

Concomitant with this research, interaction analysis

should be used as a training technique. These systems have a range of versatility that spans initial to final stages of training. Clinicians not yet enrolled in practicum can select a category system as an observational matrix, to focus observations and thus heighten awareness of therapeutic behavior. Category systems can be used by supervisors for monitoring the clinician's behavior. Finally, advanced clinicians can use these systems as tools for self-improvement. In its many uses, interaction analysis is heartily endorsed within the field of speech pathology. With research moving in this direction, significant patterns may emerge which account for at least part of the variance in clinical effectiveness.

REFERENCES CITED

Allport, G. W., Psychological models for guidance. Harvard Educ. Rev., 32, 373–381 (1962).

Anderson, H. H., The measurement of dominative and of socially integrative behavior in teachers' contacts with children. Child Dev., 10, 73–89 (1939).

Anderson, H. H., and Brewer, J. E., Studies of teachers' classroom personalities: I. Dominative and socially integrative behavior of kindergarten teachers. Appl. Psychol. Monogr. 6, Stanford University Press (1945).

Anderson, H. H., and Brewer, J. E., Studies of teachers' classroom personalities: II. Effects of teachers' dominative and integrative contacts on children's classroom behavior. Appl. Psychol. Monogr. 8, Stanford University Press (1946a).

Anderson, H. H., and Reed, M. F., Studies of teachers' classroom personalities: III. Follow-up studies of the effects of dominative and integrative contacts on children's behavior. Appl. Psychol. Monogr. 11, Stanford University Press (1946b).

Anderson, J. L., Supervision of the clinical process in speech pathology: Issues and practices. Short course presented at the American Speech and Hearing Association convention, Las Vegas (1974).

Berscheid, E., and Walster, E. H., Interpersonal Attraction. Reading, Mass.: Addison-Wesley (1969).

Blumberg, A., A system for analyzing supervisor-teacher interaction. In:

A. Simon and G. Boyer (eds.), Mirrors for Behavior. Philadelphia Research for Better Schools, Inc. (1970).

Blumberg, A., Supervisors and Teachers: A Private Cold War. Berkeley, Cal.: McCutchan Publishing Co. (1974).

Boone, D., and Goldberg, A., An experimental study of the clinical acquisition of behavioral principles of videotape self-confrontation. Final report, Project 4071, Grant OEG-8-071319-2814, Washington, D.C.: U.S. Department of Health, Education, and Welfare (1969).

Boone, D., and Prescott, T., Applications of videotape and audiotape self-confrontation procedures to training clinicians in speech and hearing therapy. Part II. Final report, Project 152310, Grant OEG-0-70-4758 (607), Washington, D.C.: U.S. Department of Health, Education, and Welfare (1971).

Boone, D., and Prescott, T., Content and sequence analysis of speech and hearing therapy. Asha, 14, 58–62 (1972).

Boone, D., and Stech, E., The development of clinical skills in speech pathology by audiotape and videotape self-confrontation. Final report, Project 1381, Grant OEG-9-071318-2814, Washington, D.C.: U.S. Department of Health, Education, and Welfare (1970).

Brown, E. L., A university's approach to improving supervision. Asha, 9, 476–479 (1967).

Byrne, D., Magnitude of positive and negative reinforcements as a determinant of attraction. J. Personal. Soc. Psychol., 2, 884–889 (1965).

Campbell, J. R., Macroanalysis: A new development for interaction analysis. J. Educ. Res., 68, 261–269 (1975).

Caple, R. B., A molar model for the training of student personnel workers. Couns. Educ. Sup., 18, 31–41 (1972).

Carkhuff, R. R., The prediction of effects of teacher-counselor training: The development of communication and discrimination selection indexes. Couns. Educ. Sup., 7, 265–272 (1969a).

Carkhuff, R. R., Helping and Human Relations: A Primer for Lay and Professional Helpers. Vols. 1 and 2. New York: Holt, Rinehart and Winston (1969b).

Carkhuff, R. R., The Development of Human Resources: Psychology, Education and Social Relations. New York: Holt, Rinehart and Winston (1971).

Carkhuff, R. R., and Berenson, B. G., Beyond Counseling and Therapy. New York: Holt, Rinehart and Winston (1967).

Carkhuff, R. R., and Truax, C. B., Toward explaining success and failure in interpersonal learning experiences. Personnel Guid. J., 44, 723–728 (1966).

Davis, G. W., An examination of dialogue and certain other factors and their influence on interaction between the client and the therapist in the therapeutic process of speech and hearing. Unpublished doctoral dissertation, Columbus: Ohio State University (1968).

Diedrich, W. M., Assessment of the clinical process. J. Kans. Speech Hear. Assoc., 1–8 (1969).

Emerick, L., and Hood, S. B., (eds.), The Client-Clinician Relationship. Springfield, Ill.: Charles C Thomas (1974).

Erickson, R., and Van Riper, C., Demonstration therapy in a university training program. Asha, 9, 33–35 (1967).

Flanders, N. A., Interaction Analysis in the Classroom: A Manual for Observers. Ann Arbor: University of Michigan (1965).

Fortune, J. C., A study of the generality of presenting behavior in teaching. Bethesda, Md.: ERIC Document Reproduction Service, ED 016 2851 (1969).

Fuller, F., Brown, O., Newlove, B., and Brown, G., Personal assessment feedback counseling for teachers. Austin, Tex.: Research and Development Center for Teacher Education, University of Texas (1973).

Fuller, F., and Manning, B., Self-confrontation reviewed: A conceptualization for video playback in teacher education. Rev. Educ. Res., 43, 197–204 (1970).

Giandomenico, A. M., Flanders' interaction analysis as a means of changing speech clinicians' verbal behavior. Unpublished doctoral dissertation, Cleveland: Case Western Reserve University (1970).

Grandstaff, H. L., A comparison of clinical behaviors of untrained, moderately trained and trained speech clinicians during articulation therapy. Unpublished doctoral dissertation, University of Cincinnati (1974).

Guildston, P., and Guildston, H., An existential approach to speech therapy. J. Commun. Disord., 5, 32–38 (1972).

Haller, R. M., Supervisor's criteria for evaluating student's performance in clinical practicum activities. Asha, 9, 479–481 (1967).

Harrison, S. L., and Carek, D. J., Psychotherapy. Boston: Little, Brown (1966).

Holland, A. L., and Matthews, J., Application of teaching machine concepts to speech pathology and audiology. Asha, 5, 474–482 (1963).

Ingram, D., and Stunden, A., Student's attitudes toward the therapeutic process. Asha, 9, 435–442 (1967).

Johnson, T., The development of a multidimensional scoring system for observing the clinical process in speech pathology. Unpublished doctoral dissertation, Lawrence: University of Kansas (1969).

Kagan, N., Multimedia in guidance and counseling. Personnel Guid. J., 49, 197–204 (1970).

Kaplan, N. R., and Dreyer, D. E., The effect of self-awareness training on student speech pathologist-client relationships. J. Commun. Disord., 7, 329–342 (1974).

Klevans, D., and Volz, H., Development of a clinical evaluation procedure. Asha, 16, 489–491 (1974).

Krumboltz, J. D., Promoting adaptive behavior: New answers to familiar questions. In: J. D. Krumboltz (ed.), Revolution in Counseling. Boston: Houghton Mifflin (1966).

Leonard, C., Gies, F., and Paden, J., The effect of selected media feedback upon the interactive behavior of student teachers. J. Educ. Res., 64, 478–480 (1971).

Lingwall, J. B., and Engmann, P., A behavioral model of the clinical process: A research, training and treatment tool. Paper presented at the American Speech and Hearing Association convention, Chicago (1971).

Lott, A. J., The potential power of liking as a factor in social change. Paper presented at the Southwestern Psychology Association meeting, Austin, Tex. (1969).

Lott, A. J., and Lott, B. E., Group cohesiveness and individual learning. J. of Educ. Psychol., 57, 61–73 (1966).

McCroskey, J. C., Larson, C. E., and Knapp, M. L., An Introduction to Interpersonal Communication. Englewood Cliffs, N.J.: Prentice-Hall (1971).

McCroskey, J. C., and McCaine, T. A., The measurement of interpersonal attraction. Speech Monogr., 41, 261–266 (1974).

MacLearie, E., Appraisal form for speech and hearing therapists. J. Speech Hear. Disord., 23, 612–614 (1958).

McReynolds, L. V., Contingencies and consequences in speech therapy. J. Speech Hear. Disord., 35, 12–24 (1970).

Marshall, W., and Hegrenes, J., Use of videotape replay. Prof. Psychol., 1, 283 (1970).

Medley, D. M., and Mitzel, H. E., Measuring classroom behavior by systematic observation. In: N. L. Gage (ed.), Handbook of Research on Teaching. Chicago: Rand McNally (1963).

Mendelsohn, G. A., and Rankin, N. O., Client-counselor compatibility and the outcome of counseling. J. Abnorm. Psychol., 74, 157–163 (1969).

Mercer, A. L., and Schubert, G. W., Nonverbal behaviors of speech pathologists in the therapy setting. Bethesda, Md.: ERIC Document Reproduction Service, ED 098-637 (1974).

Mischel, W., Personality and Assessment. New York: John Wiley & Sons (1968).

Moos, R., Sources of variance in responses to questionnaires and in behavior. J. Abnorm. Psychol., 74, 405–412 (1969).

Moos, R., Conceptualizations of human environments. Am. Psychol., 28, 652–665 (1973).

Moos, R., Ward Atmosphere Scale Manual. Palo Alto, Cal.: Consulting Psychologists Press (1974).

Mosher, R. L., and Purpel, D. E. Supervision: The Reluctant Profession. Boston: Houghton Mifflin (1972).

Mowrer, D. E., Accountability and speech therapy in the public schools. Asha, 14, 111–115 (1972).

Mowrer, D. E., An analysis of motivational techniques used in speech therapy. Asha, 16, 491–493 (1974).

Mulhern, S. T., Relationship of clinical reinforcement to spontaneous child verbalization during language training. Paper presented at the American Speech and Hearing Association convention, San Francisco (1972).

Olsen, B. D., Comparisons of sequential interaction patterns in therapy of experienced and inexperienced clinicians in the parameters of articulation, delayed language, prosody, and voice disorders. Unpublished doctoral dissertation, University of Denver (1972).

Oratio, A. R., A factor-analytic study of criteria for evaluating student clinicians in speech pathology. J. Commun. Disord., 9, 199–210 (1976a).

Oratio, A. R., The clinician's level of training as a factor in supervisors' evaluations of clinical performance. Ohio J. Speech Hear., 12, 32–38 (1976b).

Oratio, A. R., and Hood, S. B., Certain select variables as predictors of goal achievement in speech therapy. J. Commun. Disord. (in press).

Patterson, C. H., Theories of Counseling and Psychotherapy. New York: Harper & Row (1973).

Paul, G. L., Strategy of outcome research in psychotherapy. J. Consult. Psychol., 31, 109–118 (1967).

Perkins, W., Shelton, R., Studebaker, G., and Goldstein, R., The national examination in speech pathology and audiology: Philosophy and operation. Asha, 12, 175–181 (1970).

Powers, M. H., What makes an effective public school speech therapist? J. Speech Hear. Disord., 21, 461–467 (1956).

Prescott, T., The development of a methodology for describing speech therapy. Unpublished doctoral dissertation, University of Denver (1970).

Prescott, T. A., and Tesauro, P. A., A method for quantification and description of clinical interactions with aurally handicapped children. J. Speech Hear. Disord., 39, 235–243 (1974).

Rogers, E. M., and Shoemaker, F., Communication of Information. New York: The Free Press (1971).

Sapolsky, A., Effect of interpersonal relationships upon verbal conditioning. J. Abnorm. Soc. Psychol., 60, 241–246 (1960).

Schubert, G. W., and Glick, A. M., A comparison of two methods of recording and analyzing student-clinician-client interaction: ABC System and the "Boone" System. Bethesda, Md.: ERIC Document Reproduction Service, ED 098-752 (1973).

Schubert, G. W., and Laird, B. A., The length of time necessary to obtain a representative sample of clinician-client interaction. J. Natl. Student Speech Hear. Assoc., 3, 26–32 (1975).

Schubert, G. W., Miner, A., and Prather, E., A comparison of student clinicians' behaviors as measured by the analysis of behaviors of clinicians (ABC) system. Paper presented at the American Speech and Hearing Association convention, San Francisco (1972).

Schubert, G., Miner, A., and Till, J. A., The analysis of behavior of clinicians (ABC) system. Grand Forks, N.D.: University of North Dakota (1973).

Schriberg, L. D., Filley, F. S., Hayes, D. M., Kwiatkowski, J., Schatz, J. A., Simmons, K. M., and Smith, M. E., The Wisconsin procedure for appraisal of clinical competence (W-Pacc): Model and data. Asha, 17, 158–165 (1975).

Simon, A., and Boyer, E., Mirrors for Behavior: An Anthology of Observation Instruments. Philadelphia Research for Better Schools Inc. (1967).

Soloman, G., and MacDonald, F., Pretest and posttest reaction to self-viewing one's teaching. J. Educ. Psychol., 61, 280–286 (1970).

Spriestersbach, D., As I see it—clinician: A status title. Asha, 7, 464 (1965).

Sprinthall, N., Whiteley, J., and Mosher, R., A study of teacher effectiveness. J. Teach. Educ., 18, 93–106 (1966).

Stech, E. L., An empirical study of videotape self-confrontation, self-evaluation, and behavior change in speech therapist trainees. Unpublished doctoral dissertation, University of Denver (1969).

Strupp, H. H., and Bergin, A. E., Some empirical and conceptual bases for coordinated research in psychotherapy: A review of issues, trends and evidence. Int. J. Psychiatr., 7, 18–90 (1969).

Stunden, A. A., Computer simulation of therapy—the client-clinician match. Asha, 8, 100–104 (1966).

Truax, C. B., An approach to counselor education. Couns. Educ. Sup., 10, 4–15 (1970).

Truax, C. B., and Carkhuff, R. R., The experimental manipulation of therapeutic conditions. J. Consult. Psychol., 29, 119–124 (1965).

Truax, C. B., and Carkhuff, R. R., Toward Effective Counseling and Psychotherapy: Training and Practice. Chicago: Aldine (1967).

Truax, C. B., and Mitchell, K. M., Research on certain therapeutic skills in relation to process and outcome. In: A. Bergin and S. Garfield (eds.), Handbook of Psychotherapy and Behavior Change. New York: John Wiley & Sons (1970).

Turton, L. J. (ed.), Proceedings of a Workshop on Supervision in Speech Pathology. Ann Arbor: University of Michigan Press (1973).

Van Hattum, R. J., The defensive speech clinician in the schools. J. Speech Hear. Disord., 31, 234–240 (1966).

Van Riper, C., Supervision of clinical practice. Asha, 7, 75–77 (1965).

Van Riper, C., Success and failure in speech therapy. J. Speech Hear. Disord., 31, 276–279 (1966).

Van Riper, C., The stutterer's clinician. In: J. Eisenson (ed.), Stuttering: A Second Symposium. New York: Harper & Row (1975).

Wallen, J., Relationship between teaching characteristics and student behavior. Bethesda, Md.: ERIC Document Reproduction Service, ED 010-390 (1969).

Ward, L., and Webster, E., The training of clinical personnel: II. A concept of clinical preparation. Asha, 7, 103–106 (1965).

Weller, R. H., An observational system for analyzing clinical supervision of teachers. Unpublished doctoral dissertation, Cambridge, Mass.: Harvard University (1969).

Withall, J., The development of a climate index. J. Educ. Res., 45, 93–99 (1951).

Wolfe, R., The measurement of environments. In: A. Apastasi (ed.), Testing Problems in Perspective. Washington, D.C.: American Council on Education (1966).

Young, D., and Young, D. B., Individually prescribed supervisory training protocols based on a comprehensive analysis of a trainee's conference. Bethesda, Md.: ERIC Document Reproduction Service, ED 049-177 (1971).

Studies in the fields of counseling, education, and speech pathol-ogy have generally shown supervisory interactive behavior to be incon-sistent with perceptions of facilitatory communications.

chapter 4
SUPERVISOR AND CLINICIAN: An Interactive Synthesis

The previous chapter focused on the clinician's movement through the training program and his professional develop-ment. Some of the psychological difficulties in becoming a clinician were discussed, along with clinician-client interactive behavior. This chapter emphasizes the complicated interplay of interaction during the supervisor-supervisee encounter.

THE SUPERVISORY ENCOUNTER

The supervisory encounter involves both a "challenge" and a "threat" to the professional autonomy and independence of the clinician. Clinical learning means acknowledging super-visory authority and usually accepting advice and direction. Kadushin (1968), from the field of sociology, has indicated that such a dependent situation in and of itself implies an admission of ignorance and perhaps an exposure to criticism. In addition, the clinician may feel incapable of attaining the clinical standards that the supervisor has set forth. The obvious result here may be disapproval. Since the parameters of the clinical self are interrelated, anxiety evolves not only from ineptitude in clinical performance but from perceived inadequacies of self. The clinician's awareness of the supervisor's evaluative role poses still further threats.

These are but a few of the obvious difficulties intended to highlight the fact that the supervisory encounter is conceived of as much more than merely two people, supervisor and clinician, coming together to discuss protocol and management of a particular case. The supervisor is an authority figure in that he represents the academic system and, therefore, sets the tone and structure of the supervisory conference. His behaviors transmit social and emotional messages that construct a particular kind of conference climate to which the clinician must attend. From the viewpoint of education, Blumberg (1974) has given much attention to this issue:

> When a supervisor and teacher meet, the two of them form a temporary, miniature social system. It is not simply a matter of two people meeting to solve a problem, nice as that situation might be to contemplate. It is not an egalitarian situation. It is not free from authority, power, or influence. What actually occurs is that two role holders meet and one of them, typically, is the control figure by virtue of his wisdom or of his authority and power (p. 43).

Communication theorists have shown that increased conformity to demands (Critchlow, Herrup, and Dabbs, 1968), decreased fluency (Collaros and Anderson, 1969), inhibited motor responses (Doob and Gross, 1968), and altered language styles (Cowan et al., 1967) occur on the part of low status persons when confronted by perceived high status individuals. The clinician screens the supervisor's interactive tone through his individual perceptions, needs, and expectations. Parallel to the status relationships within the clinician-client dyad, the supervisor's status and power alone may significantly influence the interactive performance of a lower status individual (clinician or client). It is imperative to maintain a phenomenological or perceptual view of the supervisory encounter, because in many ways how an individual perceives the status and behavior of the supervisor is more important than these actual features themselves.

RESEARCH ON THE PERCEPTION OF SUPERVISORY BEHAVIOR

A number of studies involving the perception of supervisory interaction have emerged from the field of education. Although the majority of these studies are admittedly limited to the communications between supervisors and teachers, they have implications for the process of supervision in general.

In a classic study of interaction between supervisors and teachers, Blumberg and Amidon (1965) studied teachers' perceptions of supervisory interaction. The major questions posed by the study involved: 1) would teachers be able to discriminate various types of behavior engaged in by their supervisors, or would they instead describe supervisory behavior homogeneously?; and 2) if teachers could discriminate various supervisory interactive styles, would their differing perceptions be related to their evaluation of productivity of the conference? In order to ascertain perceptions systematically, a rating scale was used based on direct and indirect interactive dimensions (Flanders, 1960) and was administered to 166 teachers. Direct supervisory interaction was defined operationally as, "giving information or opinion, giving directions or commands, and criticizing," while indirect supervisory behavior was defined as, "accepting feelings, praising

and encouraging, accepting ideas, and asking questions."
Based on data analyses, teachers perceived four overlapping
supervisory interactive styles:

A. High direct—high indirect: The teacher sees the super-
    visor as emphasizing both direct and indirect behavior:
    he tells and criticizes but also asks and listens.
B. High direct—low indirect: The teacher perceives the
    supervisor as doing a great deal of talking and cri-
    ticizing and little asking, accepting, or encouraging.
C. Low direct—high indirect: The supervisor's interaction
    is rarely direct (telling, criticizing, and so on); emphasis
    is placed on asking, listening, and reflecting teachers'
    ideas and feelings.
D. Low direct—low indirect: The teacher sees the super-
    visor as passive, perhaps not doing much of anything.

The emergence of these categories served to answer the
first question posed by the researchers; supervisory interactive styles were not perceived on a unidimensional continuum but rather as being multidimensional. Second,
teachers felt that the supervisory conference was most productive when the supervisor was perceived as using a combination of both indirect and direct styles (styles C and A).
Teachers felt they learned more about themselves when the
supervisor was perceived as engaging in predominantly indirect interactive behavior (style C). Styles B and D seemed
to provide the teacher with relatively little learning.

In further analyses of teachers' perceptions, the researchers correlated perceived supervisory style with communicative supportiveness/defensiveness (Gibb, 1969). Teacher
defensiveness was found to be clearly related to interactive
style B. Teachers who described their supervisors as predominantly high direct—low indirect said they saw the communicative climate as focusing on control, strategy, superiority,

certainty, and evaluation. Most empathy and supportiveness developed under style C (low direct—high indirect).

In summary, teachers seemed to be saying that when their supervisors' interactive style was primarily indirect or indirect and direct, their interactions were productive, supportive, and aided learning. When the supervisor remained passive or used a predominantly direct interactive style, the conference was relatively unproductive, defense inducing, and one in which little learning took place.

In a later study, Blumberg (1968) pursued the question of interpersonal relations between supervisors and teachers. The major hypothesis in this study was whether differential perceptions of supervisory interactive styles produced differential perceptions of the interpersonal relationship between supervisors and teachers. Two instruments were used to measure interpersonal relationships, the Relationship Inventory (Barrett-Leonard, 1962) and the Teacher Perceptions of Supervisor-Teacher Interaction Scale, developed by Blumberg. The subjects for the study consisted of 210 teachers. Results led the researcher to conclude that differential perceptions of supervisory interactive styles produce differential perceptions of the state of the interpersonal relationship between teachers and supervisors. Interactive styles perceived as indirect were related to more positive interpersonal relations. Less positive and even negative interpersonal relationships were indicated by teachers when their supervisors were perceived as emphasizing styles B (high direct—low indirect) and D (Low direct—low indirect).

Blumberg and Weber (1968) studied teacher morale as a function of perceived supervisory interactive style. The same population of subjects was used as those involved in the research on interpersonal relations. High and low morale scores on a sentence completion test (Suehr, 1962) were related to perceived supervisory interactive style. The highest morale scores occurred under interactive style C (low direct—

high indirect), followed by styles A, B, and D. Supervisory styles with a strong emphasis on perceived indirectness seemed to be related to higher teacher morale.

More recently, Sanders and Merritt (1974) studied the relationship between perceived supervisory interactive style and teacher attitudes about education. This study was also based on the four-dimensional conceptualization of indirect and direct supervisory interaction. These authors concluded that interaction styles A (high direct—high indirect) and C (low direct—high indirect) produced more favorable teacher reactions on productivity, communication, and learning scales.

In a unique attempt to integrate this body of findings in education with the supervisory process in speech pathology, Underwood (1973) attempted to describe and analyze interactions between supervisors and speech clinicians. Using the Blumberg 15-category model, Underwood sought answers to the following basic questions:

1. Can reliability be obtained in using the Blumberg model to analyze supervisor-clinician interaction?
2. How representative of the entire supervisory conference is a 5-minute random sample of interaction?
3. How do the events of supervisor-clinician conferences compare with the events of supervisor-teacher conferences?
4. How do clinician effectiveness ratings of the conferences compare with supervisor effectiveness ratings?
5. Can recurring sequential patterns be identified which are typical of conferences perceived as effective and those perceived as ineffective?

Subjects for the study included eight supervisors and 15 student clinicians who conferred regularly during one academic quarter. Supervisory conferences were limited to a total of 30 minutes, after which each subject completed a six-item Effectiveness Rating Scale. This scale classified subjects' evaluations of the conferences according to effective, average, or ineffective ratings. Three conferences with each supervisor-clinician dyad were videotaped so that a total of 45 conferences were analyzed according to the Blumberg scoring system. Results indicated the following:

1. The Blumberg system was effective in analyzing supervisor-clinician interactions; inter- and intra-judge reliability was obtained at .95 and above.
2. In comparing random 5-minute samples of interaction, with total interactions of the entire session, correlation coefficients ranged from .59 to .89 with a median of .79.
3. Only one of 14 criteria was a differentiating factor in comparing events of supervisor-clinician conferences with the events of supervisor-teacher conferences.
4. Effectiveness ratings of supervisors and clinicians were very similar.
5. Effective and ineffective conferences were characterized by the following:

   Effective conferences:
   a. More clinician talk.
   b. High percentages of using clinician ideas, asking opinion, and asking for suggestions.
   c. No direct criticism.
   d. More supervisor reflection and extending understanding of clinician ideas.

   Ineffective conferences:
   a. More supervisor talk than clinician talk.
   b. A high percentage of giving information.
   c. Low percentages of accepting feelings, ideas, asking for opinions and suggestions.
   d. Use of criticism.

Underwood concluded that conferences were perceived as more effective when the clinician was encouraged to express opinions and ideas and to discover possible solutions to problems. Effective conferences were characterized by periods of silence which were followed by clinician talk rather than supervisor talk. It appeared that students needed these silent periods in order to integrate what was said and to search for solutions and alternatives. Conferences judged as ineffective consisted of the supervisor's exchange of factual information and lecturing. Underwood stated that perhaps these sessions were perceived as ineffective because little problem-solving behavior was taking place. This study seems to indicate that literature on educational supervision may have application to the process of clinical supervision in speech pathology.

IMPLICATIONS OF FINDINGS

Taken as a group, these studies lend support to the notion that supervisory interactive style has a strong influence on the process and interpersonal environment encountered in clinical supervision. It appears that in all instances an indirect supervisory interactive style consisting of listening, asking, reflecting, accepting, encouraging, and praising contributes to the supervisee's learning about himself, his feeling of being supported by the supervisor, his feeling of morale, and a positive interpersonal relationship between himself and the supervisor. It appears that this interactive approach is perceived as an effective approach to interaction within the supervisory encounter in speech pathology. Research is needed to substantiate whether clinicians transfer learning from the supervisory conference by providing effective therapy for the clients with whom they work. It is necessary to examine the influence of supervisory interactions on therapeutic performance.

To investigate this question, using a within subjects research design with repeated measures (Oratio, 1975), supervisory interactions were experimentally manipulated during conferences with eight speech clinicians over a 10-week period of clinical training. Clinicians were divided into two groups. Group 1 received high levels of supervisory inter-action on four dimensions (empathy, positive regard, con-creteness, and genuineness) during the first 5 weeks of therapy, while group 2 received low levels of interaction during that time span. During the second 5-week period, the supervisory interactive styles were reversed for both groups. The Boone-Prescott Interaction Analysis System was used to analyze the clinicians' therapy over the 10-week training period. It was found that all clinicians performed better in therapy (however, not significantly better) during the time period that they received high level supervisory interaction. When given this treatment, clinicians obtained more correct responses from their clients, and socialization for both the clinicians and clients was reduced. In addition, clinicians perceived the high level conferences as more effective, ac-cording to ratings on an effectiveness rating scale.

The most extensive study to date (Caracciolo, 1976) of the relationship between supervisory interaction and clinical effectiveness utilized 40 student clinicians and eight super-visors over a 16-week period of clinical training. Pre- and post-measures were taken from both supervisors and clini-cians on variables related to the quality of the interpersonal relationship between supervisors and clinicians and on ratings of clinical effectiveness. In addition, clinicians evaluated themselves on the intervening variable, self-esteem, during this time period. Comparisons between pre- and post-measures indicated significant increases in the clinicians' per-ceptions of self-esteem and in supervisors' and clinicians' perceptions of clinical effectiveness. When perceptions of clinical effectiveness and the quality of interpersonal condi-tions offered were compared for both subject groups, it was found that, while their mean scores differed significantly, both groups perceived a generally positive supervisory relationship and increased clinical effectiveness. Furthermore, a relationship was found between supervisors' perceptions of the quality of the interpersonal conditions offered and the clinicians' therapeutic effectiveness.

Taken together, these two studies support the assumption that the interactive environment encountered in supervision may influence not only the clinician's perceptions but therapeutic performance as well. Clearly, the effect on clinical behavior is neither conclusive nor readily understood, and further research will be needed to substantiate the existence of this trend.

The previous research has been largely concerned with perception of supervisory interaction and those interactions which are perceived as effective by both supervisors and supervisees. An important question that remains to be answered concerns supervisors' actual interactive behavior with supervisees. The following studies emphasize this parameter.

FURTHER STUDIES OF
SUPERVISORY INTERACTION

One of the first attempts to study behavioral events of the supervisory conference was by Hatten (1965). He reported limited success in determining the relationship between temporal content, topical content, and social-emotional climate on the one hand, and the supervisors' and clinicians' evaluations of the conferences on the other. No combination of the supervisory behavior characteristics accounted for more than one-third of the variance in the participants' judgments.

Studies in the fields of counseling, education, and speech pathology have generally shown supervisory interactive behavior to be inconsistent with perceptions of facilitatory communications. From the field of education, Blumberg and Cusick (1970) examined the behavior of supervisors in conferences with teachers. Recordings were made of 50 su, visory conferences and were analyzed using Blumberg's system. Supervisors spent 45 percent of their time talking, 63 percent of which consisted of directive interaction. They used "telling" interactions four times more than "asking." They offered alternatives seven times more than they asked for them, and they verbalized little encouragement or praise. When praise was expressed, it took the form of single words or short phrases, such as "good," "fine," and so on, rather than extended comments. Similarly, Walz and Roeber (1962) have shown that the usual counselor supervisory response is cognitive and information giving, with slightly negative overtones.

From the field of speech pathology, Culatta and Seltzer (1976) analyzed taped conferences of 10 supervisor-clinician dyads over an academic term. They concluded that supervisors dominated the conference; they spoke 55 percent of the time as compared to the clinician's 43 percent. The remaining 2 percent was silence. These conferences were characterized by the clinician chiefly giving information concerning the therapeutic intervention, and the supervisor developing strategies for future remediation. Irwin (1972, 1975) found that supervisors in speech pathology dominated the supervisory conferences and that experienced and inexperienced supervisors did not differ in their interactive styles.

These supervisory behaviors appear to be inconsistent with the development of the supervisee's insight, strategy, and growth, and indicate a need for a specialized form of supervisory training.

THE CLINICIAN AS A PERSON

The difficulties involved in becoming a clinician, the concept of authority inherent in the supervisory encounter, and the studies in perception of interaction all argue that supervision must be involved with the clinician as a person. Furthermore, what the clinician is, personally, affects what he does in therapy and what clients do. The purpose of supervision as clinician development enables the trainee to develop as both a person and a clinician. In asking a clinician to change his clinical behavior he must also change, at least to some extent, what he is as a person. It has been argued that the central focus of the supervisory encounter must be the clinician and his perceptions of himself (Ward and Webster, 1965; Prather, 1967; Brown, 1967). In this way, a simultaneous under-standing of self as clinician and person is reached. This of course means that the clinician must also have theoretical knowledge concerning the client's disorder, theories of re-mediation, and necessary methods and techniques within his clinical repertoire. But the clinician's perceptions, his assumptions, and how he feels about himself all affect what he says and does with clients. Therapeutic behavior is both an intellectual and emotional expression of the self.

In order to enhance the therapeutic intervention, the supervisor must take into account the powerful contributing affects of his personality and position upon the clinician, and the clinician's personality upon the client. One of the most critical factors in determining clinical growth and develop-ment, and perhaps therapeutic potency itself, involves the interpersonal-psychological dimension. The supervisor must see himself as a facilitator of human growth and decision making, a person who helps the clinician to help himself. The supervisor must understand the process of clinical growth of the clinician and offer support to it. The clinician needs the understanding and support of his colleagues and superiors, inner convictions, and self-esteem. The supervisor holds the responsibility for structuring a climate that reduces personal fear and insecurity. Moreover, the supervisor is charged with enhancing the talent and self-confidence of each individual clinician. Given the proper environment, the clinician's potentials can achieve full expression.

The definition of both speech therapy and clinical supervision as psychological, interpersonal processes argues for the need for supervisors to work with clinicians as people. Thus it becomes extremely important that a dimension of the supervisory process be oriented in this direction. The practical consequences are that supervision is incomplete unless it can deal with the clinician as a person—his assumptions, feelings, and perceptions of himself and his clinical performance. The extensive research cited earlier indicates a high correlation between the supervisory interactive climate and perceptions of effectiveness. The critical task of supervision involves recognizing and developing the full range of facilitatory conditions under which clinicians can attain clinical expertise.

THE EFFECTIVE SUPERVISOR: SKILLS OR CREDENTIALS?

What credentials must an effective clinical supervisor hold? Perhaps more importantly, what skills must the supervisor *obtain* in order to handle the enormous responsibilities for both clinician and client growth? Five major characteristics of an effective supervisor have been recommended by the American Speech and Hearing Association (Villarreal, 1964):

1. The clinical supervisor must hold an ASHA Certificate of Clinical Competence in speech pathology or audiology.
2. The clinical supervisor must be active in clinical work and capable of effective clinical demonstration teaching.
3. The clinical supervisor should possess demonstrated competence in working with a diversity of speech and hearing problems in a variety of clinical settings.

4. The clinical supervisor must not attempt to offer supervision in cases outside his area of competence.
5. The clinical supervisor should have qualifications in terms of academic degree and experience which are appreciably higher than the level of the students he is supervising.

TWO FALLACIOUS ASSUMPTIONS

There are currently two fallacious assumptions that underlie supervision in speech pathology. The first involves the belief that to be a master clinician is to be a supervisor. Although this seems to be a reasonable notion at first, the role of the supervisor goes substantially beyond the role of the clinician. Although being a clinician is a necessary condition for being a supervisor, it is not sufficient.

The second assumption involves the notion that the Certificate of Clinical Competence (CCC) is both the prelude and equivalent of supervisory competence. The results of surveys of supervisors cited in Chapter 1 indicate that supervisors themselves feel unprepared for the job functions they must realize. We also know that the process by which one obtains a CCC has little if anything to do with competence in the area of supervisory processes.

Schubert (1974) has suggested minimal requirements which specify training specific to the supervisory job function. These requirements are:

1. A master's degree in the subject area in which supervision will be administered.
2. Certificate of Clinical Competence in the subject area in which supervision will be administered.
3. Two hundred hours (internship) of practicum in supervision under the direction of a certified and experienced supervisor. The practicum should be with a wide

variety of clinicians (on a continuum from clinicians just beginning practicum to the graduate students about to finish practicum requirements).

4. Practicum experience as a supervisor, involving supervision of a wide range of clients with different disorders. (Note: It may be practical to certify individuals to supervise in specific areas such as stuttering, voice, cleft palate.)

5. Two years of paid professional experience following the completion of the Clinical Fellowship Years (CFY).

6. Knowledge of and experience with a wide variety of diagnostic tests and instruments within the subject area or areas in which supervision is to be administered.

7. Basic knowledge in scientific methodology. Be able to plan, supervise, and evaluate systematic controlled clinical research.

8. Six hours of academic course work specifically designed to prepare students to work actively as a clinical supervisor.

SUPERVISOR AS FACILITATOR OF CLINICAL GROWTH

It was suggested earlier that the supervisor's primary objectives involve changing clinician behavior and facilitating within the clinician the development of an autonomous clinical self. Autonomy suggests clinical self-scrutiny, self-direction, the self-generation of strategies for intervention, and the exercise of mature responsibility to both the client and supportive personnel. Moreover, this view of autonomy is conceptualized as the highest level of development within the clinical training process. It is therefore one of the supervisor's major tasks to help in the facilitation of the clinician's professional identity and autonomy. The essential spirit of supervision is to help the clinician achieve and maintain an autonomous, individually unique clinical style, consistent with the interests of remediating speech disorders. To accomplish this the supervisor has but one variable he can manipulate, himself. He must behave in a helping manner. Here supervisory *skills* and *processes* must be stressed rather than credentials and experience.

The supervisor must be sufficiently objective and perceptive to distinguish between the extent to which the student clinician has displayed the supervisor's particular, personal, clinical behavior and philosophy, as contrasted with the extent that his own self-actualization has helped him develop theoretical concepts and clinical behaviors that are in harmony with the self. As Arbuckle (1964) states, clinicians hardly can be effective if they are only pale carbon copies of their supervisors. The purpose of supervision is not to train the student to imitate a master but to help him grow and determine the theoretical position which makes for his greatest effectiveness in the therapeutic encounter. When we think of the relationship between supervisor and clinician, the word which applies most accurately is neither counseling nor teaching, for both of these operations are essential to effective clinical training in speech pathology. The term which most accurately applies is *growth,* and growth occurs in a relationship which is accepting and nonthreatening. Therefore, it is essential that the supervisor also be aware of his evaluative function and convert the potential threat that it may create into motivation toward self-exploration and self-actualization. Only when the clinician can expose himself without risk can self-actualization and clinical growth and development reach its highest level.

The effective supervisor is viewed as an individual who is first a master clinician. However, he is further viewed as an individual having two essential ingredients. First, the effective supervisor is a *multi-resource person* (Henderson, 1976). He functions as an information resource, an instructional resource, a human resource, and a coordinating resource. As an information resource, he is called upon to provide materials, references, insight, and knowledge. As an instructional resource, he must demonstrate technique, give direction, assist in planning strategies of intervention, be a therapist, and serve as a model. In his role as human resource, he provides support and facilitates the process of clinical growth and self-exploration within the clinician. Finally, as a coordinating resource, he is involved in coordinating and scheduling therapy, observation, diagnosis, and counseling.

There is a second ingredient of effective supervision which is even more essential; it requires that the supervisor be a *skilled interactionist.* In his one-to-one interactions with the clinician he is part of the larger strategy of intervention, which sets the stage for the clinician to become an effective interventionist. He must become aware of the dynamics of these supervisor-clinician interactions with each of his clinicians: their effect on the clinician's growth and on the supervisor-clinician relationship. As the supervisor participates in the exchange of verbal and nonverbal interactions with the clinician, his responses allow or restrict in subtle ways the clinician's attainment of insight, strategy, skill, and in essence, clinical growth and development. In order to become a skilled interactionist the supervisor must internalize a model of human interaction that is useful in detecting from moment to moment how the interaction is proceeding. Second, he actually must utilize the principles and interactive skills necessary for enhancing the clinician's professional growth. Such a model, and its uses, are presented in the following chapter. The point to emphasize here is that, through a series of personal encounters within the practicum experience, the supervisor can facilitate optimal clinician growth through his expertise as both a multi-resource person and a skilled interactionist.

REFERENCES CITED

Arbuckle, D. S., Supervision: Learning, not counseling. J. Counsel. Psychol., 11, 90–94 (1964).

Barrett-Leonard, G., Dimensions of therapist response as causal factors in therapeutic change. Psychol. Monogr. 562, Washington, D.C.: American Psychological Association (1962).

Blumberg, A., Supervisory behavior and interpersonal relations. Educ. Admin. Q., 4, 34–45 (1968).

Blumberg, A., Supervisors and Teachers: A Private Cold War. Berkeley, Cal.: McCutchan Publishing Co. (1974).

Blumberg, A., and Amidon, E., Teacher perceptions of supervisor-teacher interaction. Admin. Notebook, 14, No. 1 (1965).

Blumberg, A., and Cusick, P., Supervisor-teacher interaction: An analysis of verbal behavior. Education, Nov., 126–134 (1970).

Blumberg, A., and Weber, W., Teacher morale as a function of perceived supervisor behavior style. J. Educ. Res., 62, 109–113 (1968).

Brown, E. J., A university's approach to improving supervision. Asha, 9, 476–479 (1967).

Caracciolo, G. L., Perceptions by speech pathology student-clinicians and supervisors of interpersonal conditions and professional growth during the supervisory contract. Unpublished doctoral dissertation, New York: Teachers College, Columbia University (1976).

Collaros, P. A., and Anderson, L. R., Effect of perceived expertness upon creativity of members of brainstorming groups. J. Appl. Psychol., 53, 159–163 (1969).

Cowan, P. A., Weber, J., Hoddinott, B. A., and Klein, J., Mean length of spoken response as a function of stimulus, experimenter, and subject. Child Dev., 38, 191–203 (1967).

Critchlow, K. F., Herrup, R., and Dabbs, J. M., Jr., Experimenter influence in a conformity situation. Psychol. Rep., 23, 408–410 (1968).

Culatta, R., and Seltzer, H., Content and sequence analysis of the supervisory session. Asha, 18, 8–12 (1976).

Doob, A. N., and Gross, A. E., Status of frustrator as an inhibitor of horn-honking responses. J. Soc. Psychol., 76, 213–218 (1968).

Flanders, N., Teacher influence—pupil attitudes and achievement. Cooperative research project 397, final report. U.S. Office of

Education. Washington, D.C.: U.S. Government Printing Office (1960).

Gibb, J., Defensive communication. J. Commun., 11, 141–148 (1969).

Hatten, J. T., A descriptive and analytical investigation of speech therapy supervisor-therapist conferences. Unpublished doctoral dissertation, Madison: University of Wisconsin (1965).

Henderson, H., Personal communication, Bowling Green State University, Bowling Green, Ohio (1976).

Irwin, R. B., Interaction analysis of verbal behaviors of supervisors and speech clinicians during microcounseling sessions. Unpublished research, Columbus: Ohio State University (1972).

Irwin, R. B., Microcounseling interviewing skills of supervisors of speech clinicians. Human Commun., 4, 5–9 (1975).

Kadushin, A., Games people play in supervision. Soc. Work, 3, 23–33 (1968).

Oratio, A. R., The differential effects of high and low level supervisory conferences on student clinicians' perceptions and performance in therapy. Unpublished research, Bowling Green, Ohio: Bowling Green State University (1975).

Prather, E. M., An approach to clinical supervision. Asha, 9, 472–473 (1967).

Sanders, J., and Merritt, D. L., Relationship between perceived supervisor style and teacher attitudes. Paper presented at the American Educational Research Association 59th annual meeting, Chicago (1974).

Schubert, G. W., Suggested minimal requirements for clinical supervisors. Asha, 16, 305 (1974).

Suehr, J., A study of morale in educational settings utilizing incomplete sentences. J. Educ. Res., 56, 75–81 (1962).

Underwood, J., Interaction analysis between the supervisor and the speech and hearing clinician. Unpublished doctoral dissertation, University of Denver (1973) (c.f. Seeley, J., dissertation abstracts).

Villarreal, J., Seminar on guidelines for supervision of clinical practicum. Washington, D.C.: American Speech and Hearing Association (1964).

Walz, G. W., and Roeber, E. C., Supervisors' reactions to a counseling interview. Couns. Educ. Sup., 11, 2–7 (1962).

Ward, L., and Webster, E., The training of clinical personnel: I. Issues in conceptualization. Asha, 7, 38–40 (1965).

*When the supervisor accepts the clinician at his level of develop-
ment, accepts his clinical perceptions, and immerses himself in the
clinician's reality, the clinician is able to seek new insights and experiment with new thoughts and behaviors in the safety of the conference
environment.*

chapter 5

A SUPERVISORY TRANSACTIONAL SYSTEM

Much information has been written specifically for the clinician in speech pathology. Within our field important clinical
theories and techniques abound. However, few systematic
methodologies exist whereby the supervisor may enhance his
professional skills. Although supervisory skills are multifaceted, numerous writers have expressed the importance of
the human encounter between supervisor and clinician as a
highly significant part of clinical training. More than 10 years
ago Ward and Webster (1965) stated that the supervisor must
"provide conditions for the continued growth of the self-
actualization of students in the series of human encounters
which constitute their academic and clinical preparation" (p.
40). And in that same year Van Riper (1965) wrote:

> It is in our personal interaction with the students we supervise that
> we are able to have our most important impact. It is in this
> situation that we turn students into clinicians (p. 75).

How can the supervisor develop himself as a skilled interactionist in order to foster clinician development? He can
utilize a descriptive system which enhances prediction and

95

control of behavior as he engages in interaction with the clinician. Conceivably, there are several systems that can be used with equal effectiveness. Ultimately, the interactions that result from the use of such systems must be validated in clinician and, more importantly, client criteria. For instance, not only must the clinician perceive the interactions as helpful, but such interactions must enable the clinician to deliver more effective therapeutic services to the client. Supervisory interaction in this context is defined as transitory, one-to-one communication with the clinician.

Despite the recognized importance of interaction between supervisor and clinician, to date there are only two category systems which have been constructed and used specifically for analyzing transactions within the speech pathology supervisory conference setting (Underwood, 1974; Culatta and Seltzer, 1976). In an effort to develop and further a systematic understanding of the interactive world of the clinician and supervisor, a third system is herein presented.

This interaction system has been included for a number of reasons. First, there has been a paucity of work in this area. Second, in the surveys previously discussed, supervisors have expressed a need for a form of specialized supervisory training. Third, the literature indicates that interpersonal transactions may be critical in determining clinical growth and development and that self-confrontation procedures are an effective means of changing behavior. Finally, the system reported here incorporates a number of unique features which include the following:

1. Major elements of the system retain statistical support which validates their inclusion as categories in such a system.
2. The system is qualitative as well as quantitative and provides separate means of scoring both of these components.

3. Categories have been clustered according to the major interactive function of both the supervisor and the clinician. Each cluster thereby can be inspected for level of functioning.
4. The categories function as a guide in enabling the supervisor to achieve the two major goals of clinical supervision, developing clinician autonomy and enhancing behavioral change.
5. Since interactive events proceed over time, a temporal element has been included for time-based scoring.

NATURE OF THE TRANSACTIVE SYSTEM

The system itself contains 11 categories, seven concerned with supervisor interaction and four concerned with clinician interaction (Table 2). These dimensions are adaptations from the research of Carkhuff and his co-workers in the field of counselor education, and Culatta and Seltzer (1976) from speech pathology. Meux (1967) apprises supervisors that

Table 2. Categories and category numbers of the transactive system

Category number	Category title
Supervisor	
1	Empathy
2	Positive regard
3	Genuineness
4	Concreteness
5	Observation/information
6	Problem identification
7	Strategy
Clinician	
8	Observation/information
9	Clinical self-exploration
10	Problem identification
11	Strategy

combining categories from previously existing systems aids the identification of novel interactive behavior which is maximally effective. This strategy underlies the development of the present system.

Categories 1 through 4 (empathy, positive regard, genuineness, and concreteness) are dimensions which are shared by all human interactive processes. These dimensions set the climate for growth, development, and insight. More importantly, these dimensions retain imposing statistical support for their effects on a variety of outcome criteria, including changes on social-emotional indexes (Truax and Carkhuff, 1964, 1966; Carkhuff, 1967), as well as changes in intellective indexes, such as achievement (Aspy, 1967a, 1967b, 1967c). There is evidence to suggest that from 20 to 50 percent of the variability on these growth indexes can be accounted for by these first four core dimensions (Truax, 1961; Truax and Carkhuff, 1966; Carkhuff and Berenson, 1967). The reader will note that these four dimensions were also included as essential core conditions of the therapeutic process discussed in Chapter 3.

Research has further established that it is the person in the superior position in an interpersonal dyad (in this case, the supervisor) who determines the level of facilitation that the second person (the clinician) receives (Truax and Carkhuff, 1963, 1964, 1965). It also has been shown that interpersonal interaction may be for better or worse; that is, communications within categories 1 through 4 can either facilitate or retard personal growth and development (Truax and Carkhuff, 1963, 1964, 1966; Carkhuff and Truax, 1966; Carkhuff, 1967). Moreover, a person's level of growth and development is related to his level of self-exploration (category 9 in the present system), which in turn is related to the interactive quality of the first four core supervisory dimensions (Truax and Carkhuff, 1966; Alexik and Carkhuff, 1967;

Carkhuff and Alexik, 1967; Holder, Carkhuff, and Berenson, 1967; Piaget, Berenson, and Carkhuff, 1967).

For these reasons, delineation of the categories is such that there is greater concentration on the supervisor, whose behavior sets the psychological climate and communicative atmosphere of the conference, and who is capable of bringing the clinician to deeper levels of clinical self-exploration and higher levels of functioning. The remaining categories within the system (categories 5, 6, 7, 8, 10, and 11) reflect whether it is the supervisor or the clinician who identifies clinical problems and provides observation, information, and strategies pertinent to therapy. When it is the supervisor who provides these data, he functions to reinforce clinician dependency and impedes the process of clinical growth and development. When the supervisor facilitates both the clinician's identification of clinical problems and his divulgence of information and clinical strategies, he lays the foundation for and initiates the process of clinician growth, decision making, and autonomy.

Since all supervisor-clinician interactions can be viewed on a continuum of facilitation, a stratification across interactive categories has been provided. What looks to be an 11-category system is actually a 33-point system (3 X 11) because behavior within each category ranges on a qualitative scale from level 3 to level 1. Across all categories, level 2 is defined as the *minimally* facilitative level of supervisor-clinician functioning. Level 3 provides the *highest* facilitatory conditions, and level 1 provides *nonfacilitatory* conditions. At level 3, the supervisor actively facilitates the clinician's discussion of clinical information, his identification of clinical problems, and his development of strategies for future intervention. At level 1, the supervisor either provides this information from his own perspective or provides no clinically relevant material. In addition, he conveys little support and acceptance for

the clinician. Examples of the differential quality of interaction at these levels are provided below.

OPERATIONAL CATEGORY DESCRIPTORS AND EXEMPLARS

Supervisor Interactions

Category 1 **EMPATHY**

Level 3

Supervisor responses which add significantly to the feelings
and expressions of the clinician, in such a way as to
accurately express feelings level(s) beyond what the clinician himself was able to express.

Level 2

Supervisor responses which are interchangable with those
of the clinician, in that they express the same affect and
meaning.

Level 1

Supervisor responses which either do not attend to or
detract significantly from the feelings and expressions of
the clinician. These responses communicate significantly
less of the clinician's feelings than the clinician has com-
municated himself.

Example 1:

Clinician: *We were working on that /s/ sound and I'm not
sure she's getting it.*

Level 3
response: *It was difficult for you to get her to produce
the /s/. Although you've tried, you're wondering where to go from here, and just how to
develop that sound. You seem a bit confused at
this point.*

Level 1

response: *Well, how's her mom doing today?*

Category 2 **POSITIVE REGARD**

Level 3

Supervisor responses which communicate deep respect and concern for the clinician's worth as a person and potential as a professional practitioner.

Level 2

Supervisor responses which communicate a positive respect and concern for the clinician's feelings, experiences, and potentials.

Level 1

Supervisor responses which communicate little respect and concern, or negative regard, for the clinician's feelings, experiences, and potentials.

Example 2:

Clinician: *I've tried a number of ways now to get her to say it.*

Level 3

response: *Although your initial attempts haven't succeeded, you're determined to find a way; that's a sign of a competent clinician.*

Level 1

response: *You'll just have to try harder. As a graduate student, you should be able to do that.*

Category 3 **GENUINENESS**

Level 3

Supervisor interactions which indicate that he is freely and deeply himself in his relationship with the clinician. He is spontaneous in his interaction and open to experiences of all types, both pleasant and unpleasant. In the event of unpleasant experiences, he employs comments constructively to open further areas of inquiry.

Level 2

Supervisor interactions which provide no discrepancy between what he verbalizes and what other cues indicate he is feeling, while also providing no positive cues to indicate really genuine responses to the clinician.

Level 1

Supervisor interactions which are unrelated to what other cues indicate he is feeling at the moment, or when his responses are genuine, they are negative in regard to the clinician and appear to have a destructive effect upon him.

Example 3:

Clinician: *What do you think I should do with her?*

Level 3

response: *I know you're wondering what I would do, but I'd rather help you try to find your own way, maybe think it out. Based on my experiences, I find that works best.*

Level 1

response: *Obviously, there are any of 50 techniques I could employ.*

Category 4 **CONCRETENESS**

Level 3

Supervisor interactions which are helpful in enabling the clinician to discuss fluently, directly, and in specific terms, experiences, feelings, and various areas of concern.

Level 2

Supervisor interactions which enable the clinician to discuss clinically relevant material specifically.

Level 1

Supervisor interactions which lead or allow discussions of clinically relevant material to be dealt with in vague and abstract terms, with anonymous generalities.

Example 4:

Clinician: *She's so active, her behavior just blocks therapy.*

Level 3

response: *When she runs around the room and won't sit in her seat, you find it difficult to achieve your goal. Is that what you mean?*

Level 1

response: *Do you think that all children her age are like that?*

Category 5   **OBSERVATION/INFORMATION**

Level 3

Supervisor interactions which are requests for the clinician to provide clinically relevant observation and information pèrtinent to the therapeutic interaction or remediation.

Level 2

Supervisor interactions which provide clinically relevant observation or information pertinent to the therapeutic interaction or remediation.

Level 1

Supervisor interactions which have no direct relationship to either the supervisory or therapeutic processes.

Example 5:

Clinician: *He seems to have a number of misarticulations besides the /s/ sound.*

Level 3
response: *Can you be a little more specific? Tell me what*
these phonemes are and the kinds of tests
you've given him.

Level 1
response: *He's so cute, isn't he?*

Category 6 **PROBLEM IDENTIFICATION**

Level 3
   Supervisor interactions which are requests for the clinician
   to identify multiple clinician/client behaviors which impede
   therapeutic progress.

Level 2
   Supervisory interactions which are requests for the clinician
   to identify a single clinician/client behavior which impedes
   therapeutic progress.

Level 1
   Supervisor interactions in which the supervisor identifies
   clinician/client behavior(s) which impede therapeutic progress.

Example 6:

   Clinician: *I'm still trying to get her to say that /s/ sound.*
   Level 3
   response: *What kinds of behaviors seem to impede her*
   ability to produce that sound?

   Level 1
   response: *As I see it, she's not attending to your produc-*
   tion; her jaw is not closed and her lips are
   spread apart.

Category 7 **STRATEGY**

Level 3
   Supervisor interactions which request that the clinician

provide multiple strategies for future therapeutic intervention.

Level 2

Supervisor interactions which request that the clinician provide a single strategy for future therapeutic intervention.

Level 1

Supervisor interactions in which the supervisor provides one or multiple strategies for future therapeutic intervention.

Example 7:

Clinician: *If I could only get her to feel the difference.*

Level 3
response: *What kinds of things might you do to develop that awareness?*

Level 1
response: *By shunting the visual modality and utilizing negative practice you could do it.*

Clinician Interactions

Category 8 OBSERVATION/INFORMATION

Level 3

Clinician interactions which provide clinically relevant observation or information pertinent to the therapeutic intervention or remediation.

Level 2

Clinician interactions which are requests for the supervisor to provide clinically relevant observation or information pertinent to the therapeutic interaction or remediation.

Level 1

Clinician interactions which have no direct relationship to either the supervisory or therapeutic process.

Example 8:

Supervisor: *What did you notice in there?*

Level 3
response: *Well, she's beginning to put her tongue toward the roof of her mouth.*

Level 1
response: *She told me she's going to her uncle's house this weekend.*

Category 9 CLINICAL SELF-EXPLORATION

Level 3

Clinician interactions which indicate active and spontaneous engagement in a connected chain of deep clinical self-exploration. New behaviors, feelings, or aspects of self, or perhaps a new perceptual base for viewing self within the therapeutic encounter, may be discovered.

Level 2

Clinician interactions which are responses to clinically relevant material which has been introduced by the supervisor and concerns the clinical self. These responses occur in a mechanical manner and are devoid of attempts to add new material or explore the significance and meaning of the material.

Level 1

Clinician interactions which indicate active evasion of clinically significant self-exploration. The clinician changes the topic or shifts the focus of attention. Thus, clinically relevant self-exploration does not take place.

Example 9:

Supervisor: *You said you thought motivating her would help?*

Level 3

response: *Yes, I've been trying a number of different things, candy, stars, stickers . . . you know what worked best? . . . praise. Maybe that's what I should do, praise her. Her whole face lights up when I praise her, and I feel better about that, too. When I praised her she seemed to work harder.*

Level 1

response: *Yeah, but I don't know, her mother says she and her brother fight a lot.*

Category 10 **PROBLEM IDENTIFICATION**

Level 3

Clinician interactions in which the clinician identifies multiple clinician/client behaviors which impede therapeutic progress.

Level 2

Clinician interactions in which the clinician identifies a single clinician/client behavior which impedes therapeutic progress.

Level 1

Clinician interactions which are requests for the supervisor to identify clinician/client behavior(s) which impede therapeutic progress.

Example 10:

Supervisor: *I wonder what behaviors you see as blocking therapy?*

Level 3

response: *Well, first, she isn't really focusing on her articulators in the mirror. She has to try to round her lips, and we also need to get carryover within the home.*

Level 1

response: *I don't know, what do you think?*

Category 11 **STRATEGY**

Level 3

Clinician interactions which provide multiple strategies for future therapeutic intervention.

Level 2

Clinician interactions which provide a single strategy for future therapeutic intervention.

Level 1

Clinician interactions which request that the supervisor provide one or multiple strategies for future therapeutic intervention or make decisions regarding future remediation.

Example 11:

Supervisor: *What kinds of things do you think would help her?*

Level 3

response: *I think next time I'll sit closer to her and show more physical contact. Then I'll use the language master and phonic mirror to blend those sounds. Also, after I praise her, I'll tell her why it was good.*

Level 1

response: *Should I use a mirror or not? What do you think?*

DELIMITING FACTORS

It should be mentioned that the categories themselves, within the system, contain delimiting factors. The most obvious concerns the high degree of subjectivity on the part of the user. Such subjectivity cannot be avoided. In actuality, the supervisory conference is a highly subjective experience. In using the instrument, emphasis has been placed upon ratings and reratings by both the same and different users, and intra- and inter-judge reliability have been obtained beyond the .05 alpha level using the binomial test (Siegel, 1956).

A second delimiting factor involves the identification of only verbal transactions by the system, and identification is limited to only those transactions which can be classified within the range of the operational definitions provided for each category. One could assume that perhaps both non-verbal and unorthodox communications taken together may significantly influence the clinician's perceptions, development, and perhaps behavioral change. However, no single system can be expected to account for all of the details of human interaction, and the categories, taken as they are, have been shown to account for a significant proportion of variance on a variety of outcome indexes. In the end, primary emphasis is placed upon mean levels of functioning for both supervisor and clinician within major interactive category clusters, as assessed by randomly selected conference excerpts. Therefore, although interaction at a particular point in the conference may be rated low, if both supervisor and clinician function at high levels throughout the majority of the conference, the overall average ratings within category clusters will be elevated. As experienced supervisors realize, there are certainly times during the conference when the supervisor is expected to take a direct interactive stance. However, the overall tone of the conference should emphasize indirect supervisor verbalizations as a means of enhancing the clinician's insight and problem-solving abilities. Based on experience in using the instrument, and the extensive research from which the categories were derived, the system emerges as a valuable training tool for the clinical supervisor in speech pathology.

SUPPORTIVE SUPERVISION AND COUNSELING

As the reader can see, the system is both a descriptive and prescriptive approach to the supervisory conference. It posits a phenomenological "clinician-centered" counseling approach to the supervisory conference. The difficulties the student is faced with in becoming a clinician, the extensive research on the perception of supervisory interaction and actual supervisory interaction, the research findings which relate the effects of these counseling dimensions to learning and behavior change, the need to address the clinician as a person, and the critical nature of supervisory interaction to the process of training all argue for and support such an approach. Moreover, as Shaplin (1961) points out in reference to student teaching, the objectives and procedures of clinical supervision as indicated resemble in many ways the process of client-centered counseling but with less emphasis upon personality reconstruction. Such similarities are summarized in the following excerpt (Shaplin, 1961):

> Examination of the appropriateness of the person's reactions and defenses, the inquiry into why things are this way, the achievement of emotional insight, and the search for new adaptive behavior congenial to the emotional growth that takes place (p. 35).

In further support, it is recognized that the clinician brings the intellectual and emotional stress caused by his practicum experience to the supervisory conference. A clinician-centered conference is attuned to the vital aspects of the clinician's personality and provides practices for facilitating growth processes. The view that self-knowledge is important to professional growth and development orients supervision toward centering on the clinician. This theory as applied to the supervisory conference emphasizes the clinician's responsibility for analysis of behavior, identification of problems, and planning of solutions. It is directly concerned with achieving greater self-knowledge by concentrating on intensive one-to-one interaction designed to effect change in individual behavior.

This approach to the supervisory conference retains a place for phenomenological and objective viewpoints within the same system. These are conceived of as necessary ingredients for supervision which orients itself toward developing clinician autonomy, growth, and behavioral change. Discussions about one's self, the actual therapeutic intervention, and the self within the encounter become an integral part of the supervisory conference.

DEFINING SUPERVISOR-CLINICIAN BEHAVIOR

Who is the clinician in such an approach? The present approach to the supervisory conference is based on the assumption that, in theory, the clinician receives concomitant instruction in the acquisition of technical skills and knowledge. (The comprehensive supervisory model presented in the following chapter confirms this assumption.) What the clinician now needs is an opportunity to focus on his clinical behavior and clinical theory and to cognitively reorganize this information for purposes of more powerful, future, therapeutic interventions. Through the structure of indirect clinician-centered interaction, the trainee is led toward self-exploration in a supportive context.

Who is the supervisor in this interactive approach? In Kopp's terms (1972), "he operates as a counter-puncher, each movement being a response to the [clinician's] words, gestures, or postures" (p. 18). To the degree that the supervisor is able to interact with the clinician at high levels, the clinician will become more self-directing, more autonomous, more confident, and more similar to the kind of clinician he needs to be. When the supervisor accepts the clinician at his level of development, accepts his clinical perceptions, and immerses himself in the clinician's reality, the clinician is able to seek new insights and experiment with new thoughts and behaviors in the safety of the conference environment. When the supervisor is evaluative and dogmatic and imposes his clinical style upon the clinician, the clinician's self-actualization, growth, and autonomy are stifled, and both resistance to the dependency upon the supervisor become increased. The Sufi Teaching-Story of the Water-Melon Hunter (Kopp, 1972) best illustrates this point:

> Once upon a time there was a man who strayed from his own country into the world known as the Land of Fools. He soon saw a number of people flying in terror from a field where they had been trying to reap wheat. "There is a monster in that field," they told him. He looked and saw that it was a water-melon.
>
> He offered to kill the "monster" for them. When he had cut the melon from its stalk, he took a slice and began to eat it. The people became even more terrified of him than they had been of the melon. They drove him away with pitchforks, crying, "He will kill us next, unless we get rid of him."
>
> It so happened that at another time another man also strayed into the Land of Fools, and the same thing started to happen to him. But, instead of offering to help them with the "monster," he agreed with them that it must be dangerous, and by tiptoeing away from it with them he gained their confidence. He spent a long time with them in their houses until he could teach them, little by little, the basic facts which would enable them not only to lose their fear of melons, but even to cultivate them themselves (p. 8.)*

INSTRUCTIONAL PROCEDURES FOR USING THE SYSTEM

The system is designed to enable supervisors to categorize conference transactions and to develop insight into the level at which they and their clinicians function. Again, it should be pointed out that the clinician's ability to explore himself in relation to his execution of therapeutic procedures, his

---

*From **The Way of the Sufi** by Indries Shah. Reprinted by permission of Curtis Brown, Ltd., and by the publisher, E. P. Dutton & Co. Copyright ©1968 by Indries Shah. No part of the work reprinted herein may be reproduced without the express written permission from the Author's agent, Curtis Brown, Ltd., New York, N.Y., and from E. P. Dutton & Co., New York, N.Y.

ability to identify problems which impede therapeutic progress, and his ability to devise and invent strategies for future remediation are the central focus of the supervisory conference. The effectiveness or ineffectiveness of the conference is in large part determined by the mean levels of functioning of both the supervisor and the clincian. By virtue of his position, the supervisor must accept the role as controller and influencer of the conference transactions.

Recording

The first step in capturing the interaction which transpires during the conference involves making a tape recording of the entire supervisory conference. After the conference is completed, the supervisor replays the tape and randomly selects a 5-minute excerpt for scoring. (He may wish to transcribe the excerpt to ensure accuracy of scoring.) The scoring is done on the Score Sheet (see pages 122–123).

Scoring

Each box on the Score Sheet represents 3 seconds on the horizontal axis and both level and type of interaction on the vertical axis. The supervisor listens to the first interaction and places a horizontal mark (−) across the center of the first box on the Score Sheet corresponding to that interaction. Every 3 seconds he places a mark in a box within the next row which corresponds to the interaction. The supervisor may want to stop the tape frequently (or consult his transcript if he is using one) in order to be certain of the accuracy of his scoring. The following are a list of ground rules for continuous scoring:

1. Select a random 5-minute excerpt from the middle of the conference. Initial and final 5-minute segments of the conference should not be selected for analysis. Experience in using the system suggests that the interaction within a randomly selected 5-minute excerpt

selected from the middle portion of the conference is highly representative of the total conference inter-action.

2. Score interactions every 3 seconds. If more than one interactive event occurs during the 3-second interval, then all events within that interval should be scored.

3. Each change in an interaction should be scored. For example, if the interaction moves from "problem iden-tification" to "strategy," or supervisor interaction is followed by clinician interaction, each change should be scored. If no change occurs after the 3-second in-terval, score the previous category.

4. The use of "Um hum" by the supervisor is interpreted as a verbal lubricant and therefore is scored in category 4, at level 2. As a clinician interaction, it is scored in category 9, at level 2.

5. Approximately 100 boxes should be marked, designating that 100 interactions have been categorized.

When scoring is completed, each horizontal mark should be connected, forming a graphic illustration of the con-ference transaction. Finally, the graph should be scanned horizontally and interactions at each level within each cate-gory should be totaled and indicated under the "Totals" column at the right of the graph.

Transferring and Analyzing Data

The following are guidelines for transferring interactive data from the Score Sheet to the Analysis Sheet (see pages 124–125):

1. Add the total number of interactions within each cate-gory, for each of the 11 categories. Indicate that total under "Number of events" on the Analysis Sheet.

2. Within each category, multiply the number of inter-active events at each level by the level at which these

interactions were scored. Total these products in each category and indicate their sum under "Effectiveness levels" on the Analysis Sheet.

3. Since each box on the Score Sheet represents a 3-second time interval, multiply the total number of events on the Analysis Sheet by three and indicate the product for each category under the heading "Time."

4. Obtain totals for "Events," "Effectiveness levels," and "Time" by adding the data within each of the four major category clusters.

5. Obtain indexes for each of the four category clusters by placing the total from the "Effectiveness levels" over the "Events" total and dividing. The index is the mean level of functioning within each category cluster.

6. Obtain supervisor and clinician totals by transferring "Event totals" and "Time totals," under the appropriate headings, to the bottom of the analysis sheet.

7. Calculate the grand mean of the four category-cluster indexes. This mean represents the composite of all categories. Based on this number, assign to the conference a molar evaluation from 1 to 3 and indicate any comments at the bottom of the Analysis Sheet.

SAMPLE CONFERENCE

The following is an actual conference excerpt, scored and analyzed according to the above procedures. After becoming familiar with the procedures, the reader may want to cover the category classifications (on the lefthand column of the transcript) in order to test his ability to use the system.

(Category: level)

Clinician

(8:3) Anyway, with that /s/ sound, she is putting her tongue toward the roof of her mouth, so at least she's getting a new tongue position.

Supervisor

(4:2) Um hum.

Clinician

(8:3) And today we worked on putting the sound in syllables, like *say, see, sai,* and she could do that.
       And then I started working on words, and it will take her like three or four times and then she'll do it.

Supervisor

(1:2) She can produce the sound in syllables, as well as in words, but words seem to give her a little more trouble.

Clinician

(8:3) Yes, that's right, but now instead of having her just say words, I'm having her put articles before the words, like "the sun," to try to get it into more of a conversational thing, you know, 'cause when you talk you don't say "sun," you always say "the sun."

Supervisor

(4:2) Um hum.

Clinician

(8:3) So we were working on that and that was really good, because before, anytime she said "the sun," she always said "nun," she never said /s/ at all.

Supervisor

(1:3) Here, she used to omit the sound completely, and now you've gotten her to not only produce the sound in syllables and words but also in some two-word utterances and you feel pretty good about that in terms of your own clinical skills. You kind of think you'd like to continue along that same track with her.

Clinician

(11:2) Yes, I would, that's basically what I'm going to work on with her next time; I'm just going to put articles before that, and maybe we'll get into phrases.

(9:2) Then I don't know if I should do /g/ or not. I think I can, because she's worked on that before.

(11:1) Or do you think I should just forget about that?

Supervisor

(1:3)   You want to do the best you can for her, in getting her to speak as intelligibly as possible over a short period of time.

(2:3)   And you certainly have the skill to enable her to master both of those sounds this quarter.

(1:2)   But you're not quite sure if you should try it, is that right?

Clinician

(9:2)   Yes, like I don't know, I want her . . . , I don't know what I should do, you know.

(11:1) Do you have any opinion?

Supervisor

(1:2)   You kind of feel like you . . .

Clinician

(9:2)   I don't know if I'm going to confuse her.

(8:3)   Because Anne's not really a smart kid, she's kind of, I hate to say low intelligence, but it takes her a while to pick up what you're talking about.

Supervisor

(4:2)   Um hum.

Clinician

(8:3)   Like I asked her to put something in a sentence, and she didn't even know what a sentence was.

(9:2)   And it seems to me that other 5-year-old children I had worked with had no problem doing that.

Supervisor

(3:3)   I feel almost a sense of despair in what you say.

Clinician

(8:3)   Yeah, and she was just at a total loss to put the word in a sentence. And then just that one day when we were working on the /g/, you walked in the therapy room and said, "Anne, what are you working on?" And she said /s/, and we'd been working on the /g/ the whole therapy.

(9:2)   So now I don't know whether she's getting confused and I should just forget that and keep on the /s/ like before.

Supervisor

(1:3)   You don't want to confuse her, 'cause she may not be as bright as some of the other children you've worked with, but yet you would like to develop both sounds.

(7:2) I wonder how you might get her to concentrate on both of those sounds, more so than she has in the past?

Clinician

(10:2) Motivation—I think I need to find other ways to get her really motivated.

Supervisor

(1:2) You think if you could motivate her, her attention on her sounds would be better.

Clinician

(9:2) Yes, like I've been trying different things. Like one day I tried stickers, and another day I tried stars. I even tried candy with her.

(9:3) You know what worked best? When I praised her. You could just see how happy that made her when I told her how well she was doing; her whole face lit up. Maybe that's what I should do, give her more praise.

(11:2) That's what I'll do next time, give her plenty of praise and tell her why I'm praising her.

Supervisor

(2:3) That sounds like a good idea. I knew you could find a solution.

(7:2) Now, I wonder how else we could help Anne to pay closer attention and produce these sounds? You said you think she needs motivation, but maybe . . .

Clinician

(10:2) I don't think her mom's working with her. I think she just knows that if she doesn't do it her mother's just going to say, "Now Anne, I wish you'd get that tongue up." 'Cause that's the way the mother acts toward her in the clinic.

Supervisor

(1:2) It sounds like you're a bit upset by that, and you'd like to get her mom more involved.

Clinician

(10:2) Yeah, Anne's been coming now for her third quarter and she still hasn't improved.

(9:3)   You know what might be good? Maybe I could just say something to the mom, like, "Why don't you try working with her a little more?" Say it in kind of a subtle way. I don't know, it's kind of hard. You don't want parents to get personally affronted. "Why don't you try working with her more?" (harsh tone, jokingly)

Supervisor

(1:2)   Think if you mention that to her mom there's a possibility she'd take it the wrong way, but yet you feel we need her help. You want to be careful but . . .

Clinician

(8:3)   Yeah, her mother's not an easy person to deal with.

(9:3)   I wonder if her mother knows how to work with her; I don't think she would know.

You know what might be good. Maybe I could bring the mother into the session and do therapy for a half hour, then show her mom how to do it. Yeah, and I could watch her work with her. Maybe I could do that, just thought of that.

(11:3) Maybe next week I'll have the mom come in and observe me and then I'll have her work with Anne for the last 15 minutes.

Supervisor

(1:2)   Kind of have the mother do therapy with Anne.

Clinician

(11:3) Yeah, and than I'll just see what she's doing at home with her and I'll help her to work with her. And I can compare what she's getting from her mother with what she's getting from me.

Supervisor

(2:2)   I like that idea; that sounds real good.

Clinician

(9:2)   Well, that's basically it. Why, I think I just solved my own problem. That's what I'll do.

Supervisor

(4:2)   What did you say?

Clinician

(9:2)   I said I just solved one of my own problems right now. I just found something I could do that will make it work out.

DATA INTERPRETATION

When we examine the scoring and analysis sheets for this sample conference, a substantial portion of information becomes evident. Inspection of the supervisor's and clinician's total talking time shows that during this 4½-minute segment the clinician talked more than twice as long as the supervisor. Of the total number of interactive events, 63 were clinician events and 30 were supervisor events.

In analyzing clinician interaction, we see that the majority of clinician verbalizations were introspective (44 out of 63 interactions). During this time the clinician functioned at an extremely high level, indicated by a mean index of 2.68. In addition, a significant portion of high level strategy interaction occurred as evidenced by a mean index of 2.21. Because level 3 is defined as the maximal facilitatory level, these overall clinician interactive levels appear quite impressive.

In analyzing supervisor interaction, we can see from inspection of category clusters that the vast majority of supervisory interactions (25 out of 30 interactions) were spent in building a facilitatory conference climate. In this dimension, the supervisor was quite successful, as evidenced by his conference climate index of 2.40, substantially above the minimal level of facilitation. Such a climate obviously facilitated the high interactive levels achieved by the clinician. Few supervisor interactions were spent in directly facilitating clinician growth (five out of 30 interactions), although even in this dimension the supervisor functioned at the minimal facilitatory index level of 2. Perusal of supervisory interactive data indicates that the supervisor's major strength was in developing a conference climate conducive to clinician introspection and strategy. The conference was generally positive, as evidenced by these data, and worthy of a molar evaluation of 2.32.

As with any system developed for analyzing human interaction, the present one contains delimiting factors and is admittedly incomplete. The major thrust of the system is simply to enable supervisors to reliably determine supervisor-clinician levels of interactive functioning. For this purpose the system emerges as a valuable supervisory tool.

Score Sheet

Supervisor: Date:

Clinician: Length of
              Conference:

Legend

Each |—| = 3 seconds

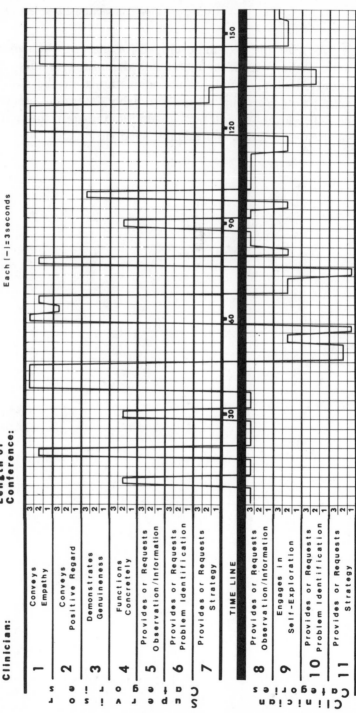

Supervisor Categories

1   Conveys Empathy

2   Conveys Positive Regard

3   Demonstrates Genuineness

4   Functions Concretely

5   Provides or Requests Observation/Information

6   Provides or Requests Problem Identification

7   Provides or Requests Strategy

TIME LINE

Clinician Categories

8   Provides or Requests Observation/Information

9   Engages in Self-Exploration

10   Provides or Requests Problem Identification

11   Provides or Requests Strategy

Totals

		Totals
1	Conveys Empathy	7 / 10
2	Conveys Positive Regard	2 / 1
3	Demonstrates Genuineness	1
4	Functions Concretely	4
5	Provides or Requests Observation/Information	
6	Provides or Requests Problem Identification	
7	Provides or Requests Strategy	5

TIME LINE

8	Provides or Requests Observation/Information	17
9	Engages in Self-Exploration	13 / 14
10	Provides or Requests Problem Identification	7
11	Provides or Requests Strategy	6 / 4 / 2

Supervisor Categories

Clinician Categories

180   210   240   270   300

ANALYSIS SHEET

Supervisor: _____ Clinician: _____ Date: _____ Length of conference: _____

Supervisor category counts

Conference climate categories	Number of events	Effectiveness levels	Time
1	17	41	51
2	3	8	9
3	1	3	3
4	4	8	12

CC total 25   EL1= 60   STT1= 75´

$\dfrac{\text{EL total}}{\text{CC total}} = 60/25 = 2.40$ $\overline{X}$ = Conference climate index

Clinician category counts

Clinician introspection categories	Number of events	Effectiveness levels	Time
8	17	51	51
9	27	67	81

CI total 44   EL1= 118   CTT1= 132

$\dfrac{\text{EL total}}{\text{CI total}} = 118/44 = 2.68$ $\overline{X}$ = Clinician introspection index

Growth facilitation categories	Number of events	Effectiveness levels	Time
5			
6			
7	5	10	16
GF total	5 EL2= 10		STT2= 16

$\dfrac{\text{EL total}}{\text{GF total}} = 10/5 = 2 \quad \bar{X} =$ Growth facilitation index

Strategy intervention categories	Number of events	Effectiveness levels	Time
10	7	14	21
11	12	27	36
SI total	19	42	57
	EL2= 42		CTT2= 57

$\dfrac{\text{EL total}}{\text{SI total}} = 42/19 = 2.21 \quad \bar{X} =$ Strategy intervention index

Supervisor totals

CC total + GF total = Event total   30

STT1 + STT2 = Time total   90

Clinician totals

CI total + SI total = Event total   63

CTT1 + CTT2 = Time total   189

Molar conference evaluation

Conference effectiveness: 2.32

Lo   Hi

1   1.5   2   2.5   3

Comments:

REFERENCES CITED

Alexik, M., and Carkhuff, R. R., The effects of the manipulation of client depth of self-exploration upon high and low functioning counselors. J. Clin. Psychol., 23, 212–215 (1967).

Aspy, D., The differential effects of high and low functioning teachers upon student achievement. Unpublished manuscript, Gainesville: University of Florida (1967a).

Aspy, D., The relationship between teacher functioning on facilitative dimensions and student performance on intellective indices. Unpublished dissertation, Lexington: University of Kentucky (1967b).

Aspy, D., Counseling and education. In: R. R. Carkhuff (ed.), The Counselor's Contribution to Facilitative Processes. Urbana, Ill.: Parkinson (1967c).

Carkhuff, R. R., The Counselor's Contribution to Facilitative Processes. Urbana, Ill.: Parkinson (1967).

Carkhuff, R. R., and Alexik, M., The differential effects of the manipulation of client self-exploration upon high and low functioning therapies. J. Counsel. Psychol., 18, 218–221 (1967).

Carkhuff, R. R., and Berenson, B. G., Beyond Counseling and Therapy. New York: Holt, Rinehart and Winston (1967).

Carkhuff, R. R., and Truax, C. B., Toward explaining success and failure in interpersonal learning experiences. Personnel Guid. J., 46, 723–728 (1966).

Culatta, R., and Seltzer, H., Content and sequence analysis of the supervisory sesson. Asha, 18, 8–12 (1976).

Holder, T., Carkhuff, R. R., and Berenson, B. G., The differential effects of the manipulation of therapeutic conditions upon high and low functioning clients. J. Counsel. Psychol., 14, 63–66 (1967).

Kopp, S. B., If You Meet the Buddah on the Road, Kill Him! Palo Alto, Cal.: Science and Behavior Books (1972).

Meux, M. O., Studies of learning in the school setting. Rev. Educ. Res., 37, 539–562 (1967).

Piaget, G., Berenson, B. G., and Carkhuff, R. R., The differential effects of high and low functioning counselors upon high and low functioning clients. J. Consult. Psychol., 17, 41–45 (1967).

Shaplin, J., Practice in teaching. Harvard Educ. Rev., 31, 35 (1961).

Siegel, S., Nonparametric Statistics. New York: McGraw-Hill (1956).

Truax, C. B., The process of group psychotherapy. Psychol. Monogr., 75, No. 14 (Whole No. 511) (1961).

Truax, C. B., and Carkhuff, R. R., For better or worse: The process of psychotherapeutic personality change. In: Recent Advances in the Study of Behavior Change. Proceedings of the Academic Assembly on Clinical Psychology, sponsored by the Department of Psychiatry, McGill University, Montreal (1963).

Truax, C. B., and Carkhuff, R. R., Significant developments in psychotherapy research. In: L. E. Abt and B. F. Reiss (eds.), Progress in Clinical Psychology. New York: Grune & Stratton (1964).

Truax, C. B., and Carkhuff, R. R., The experimental manipulation of therapeutic conditions. J. Consult. Psychol., 29, 119–124 (1965).

Truax, C. B., and Carkhuff, R. R., An Introduction to Counseling and Psychotherapy: Training and Practice. Chicago: Aldine (1966).

Underwood, J., Supervision of the clinical process in speech pathology: Issues and practices. Short course presented at the American Speech and Hearing Association convention, Las Vegas (1974).

Van Riper, C., Supervision of clinical practice. Asha, 3, 75–77 (1965).

Ward, L., and Webster, E., The training of clinical personnel: I. Issues in conceptualization. Asha, 7, 38–40 (1965).

These supervisory operations take place within an intensive cycle of clinical supervision, in which the supervisor and clinician, in a colleagual relationship, function to achieve goals which are specific to clinician development.

chapter 6
A MOLAR MODEL OF CLINICAL SUPERVISION

The use of a model is frequently the most convenient way to think about the structure of a process. It attempts to establish the best way of leading to a result. In the model described here the result is a program of supervision for the preparation of professional speech clinicians. Models typically go through periods of evolution and change as more knowledge is acquired relative to the nature of a phenomenon. It is expected that this model will also undergo change, and for this reason a degree of flexibility is intended.

Few operational models have been proposed relative to the process of clinical supervision in speech pathology (Anderson, 1973; Schriberg et al., 1975; Caracciolo, 1976; Culatta, 1976). Formalization has not been achieved due to the limited knowledge and uncertainty concerning the concepts involved. Although the model presented here is admittedly incomplete, it is based on current knowledge and practice within the social and behavioral sciences. Moreover, this comprehensive approach to supervision arises out of the need to improve the clinical training process, as clearly supported in the literature (Sheehan and Martyn, 1971; Cooper,

129

1973; Culatta, Colucci, and Wiggins, 1975; Culatta and Seltzer, 1976).

ELEMENTS AND OBJECTIVES OF THE MODEL

The proposed model embraces an intensive series of training experiences which include as major elements observation, analysis, post-therapy conferencing, didactic teaching, micro-therapy, live demonstration, and actual clinical practice. Although the component of supervision is central, each element contributes to the others and ultimately to the student's understanding of both the therapeutic and the supervisory processes. The model is conceptualized as fluid and dynamic, with supervision at its core and feeding into all other components (Figure 5).

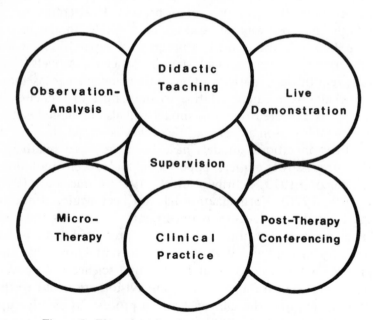

Figure 5. Elements of an integrated supervisory process.

In order to construct a model, some idea of objectives must exist. The present model encompasses first the two primary objectives of clinical supervision: changing clinician behavior in a specific direction, thus enabling the clinician to change the client's behavior in a more positive direction; and developing within the student clinician professional independence and clinical autonomy. Second, it focuses on the following clinician skill areas which have previously been discussed as critical to the clinician's professional development and effective therapeutic performance: technical knowledge, clinical skill, and self-exploration.

Within this model, the supervisory process is concerned with both cognitive and conative learning and strives to effect change in both of these dimensions. Within the model exists an obvious bias for a comprehensive, integrated process of supervision. In meeting the above objectives, the model is structured to provide experiences and skills which will take the clinician from his very entrance into clinical practicum to the final stages of clinical training. The process is structured so that the student is continuously provided with deeper experiences until he emerges as a fully functioning, self-scrutinizing professional. The supervisory functions employed to meet the above objectives are outlined in Table 3.

Table 3. Supervisory functions leading to clinical training objectives

Number	Supervisory function	Clinician objective
1	Didactic teaching	Technical knowledge
2	Clinical practice Demonstration	Clinical skill
3	Post-therapy conferencing	Self-exploration
4	Observation Analysis Micro-therapy	Behavioral change

Each of these supervisory operations takes place within an intensive cycle of clinical supervision, in which the supervisor and clinician, in a colleagual relationship, function to achieve goals which are specific to clinician development. The nature of each procedure in meeting the above objectives is discussed below.

Didactic Teaching

Technical knowledge has been formally transmitted to the student throughout his academic career. It includes facts, principles, theories, and methodologies as well as professional protocols, attitudes, and values. However, much of this information loses relevance for the student until the practicum experience provides opportunities for its use. In the student's transition from exclusive classroom learning to actual participation in clinical work, new principles and theories evolve which have application to his present situation. The supervisor has the responsibility for exposing the student, through the supervisory component of didactic teaching, to these new and previously learned theories.

Clinical Practice and Demonstration

The central experience to an effective clinical training program is supervised clinical practice. Skill within this dimension is most essential and is enhanced over time through actual clinical work. However, the transition from technical knowledge to actual use in practice is not easy. The presence of an actual model is crucial to this form of learning. Therefore, supervisory demonstration, in which the supervisor serves as a model and a guide, becomes important in many ways. In acknowledging the importance of this supervisory component. Erickson and Van Riper (1967) state:

> It has become our firm conviction that the observation of demonstration therapy is a vital part of our training program at both the

graduate and undergraduate levels. Demonstration therapy not only illustrates the textual and lecture information our students receive, but it supplements it. Attitudes, clinical judgment, role behaviors and a host of important therapy principles seem to be acquired more easily through observation and empathy, especially when these are accompanied by the clinician's commentary and when an opportunity for dialogue and discussion is made available (p. 33).

Further study of the demonstration component is needed in order to increase its effectiveness as a formal learning component within the supervisory process.

Learning by practice may be divided into three phases: observation, imitation, and internalization. Within the first phase, observation, the clinician sees that as a result of specific behaviors the clinical performance succeeds or fails. The clinician becomes familiar with these behaviors and focuses on the outcome of the client's speech behavior as well as on the observation of the model.

In the second phase, imitation, the clinician executes the behavior that he has observed in practice. Imitation of a model over an extended period of time results in a shallow "apeing" of clinical behavior; therefore, the third phase is necessary.

In the internalization phase, the clinician modifies the clinical behavior he observed and practiced, so that the behavior becomes personalized. His clinical behavior can now be differentiated from the model by its unique personal overtones.

Post-therapy Conferencing

The supervisory conference has been discussed in detail in the preceding chapter and therefore need not be reviewed at this point. It should be mentioned, however, that the fundamental purpose of the conference is to provide a time and context, immediately following therapy, in which the clinician can engage in self-exploration. Self-exploration provides opportunities for the clinician to integrate, discover, and develop aspects of his clinical personality, clinical practice, and technical knowledge. Such an opportunity leads to independence and allows the clinician to take charge of his behavior. Sherif and Sherif (1969) support the proposition that perception and judgment are not just cognitively determined but involve a combination of internal conative and external operative factors. Self-exploration helps the clinician focus on these factors. The responsibility for clinical judgment and decision making ultimately must rest with the clinician. The conference which leads the clinician into self-exploration develops this capacity.

Observation

Observation is not passive, but an active process with specific purposes. The supervisor's first job is to make a detailed record of what the clinician says and does, and what the client says and does. Here audiotape or videotape is used to capture the events of therapy. At some point while observing this replay of the session, the supervisor and clinician are confronted with the question of what to observe. In essence, this amounts to how to make sense of the therapeutic process and how to identify and categorize the events of therapeutic behavior in order to make inferences. The one criterion of therapy whose validity has not been challenged involves the response of the client. The supervisor, in judging outcome, then must emphasize the client's responses and behavior as he is engaged in therapy. What clients say and do during therapy is the most immediate and valid index of the therapeutic affect available to the supervisor. By focusing on client behavior in relation to the intent of the clinician, the supervisor and clinician have a baseline against which to gauge the results of change in both clinician and client performance.

What client behavior, then, is useful for the supervisor and clinician to look at and analyze? What client behavior is the best index of improvement? Here, the clinician's goals provide a valuable point of reference. The supervisor knows these goals from the lesson plan. Does the client work with or against the clinician? Although resistance is more often the rule in changing fixed speech habits, does client behavior impede the clinician's planned objectives? For a further discussion of this point see Emerick's conceptualization of "compatible friction" between clinician and client (Emerick and Hood, 1974).

Analysis as Behavioral Change

Speech therapy as a transactive process can be subjected to interaction analysis. This analysis of therapy requires the use of one of the many systems available to the clinician and supervisor. The analysis further requires specific skills which should be acquired by the clinician during the practicum experience. Therapeutic analysis is viewed as a rigorous, systematic, ongoing, and cooperative endeavor between clinician and supervisor. As the clinician acquires skill in the analysis of his therapy, he becomes a careful critic of his therapeutic practice independent of supervisory input.

As the supervisor and clinician engage in the analysis of therapy, they identify behaviors and patterns of behavior according to the interactive system in use. Based on this quantification and analysis, hypotheses about appropriate changes in clinical behavior are formed. Change is built on successful behavior and largely on the clinician's own abilities to analyze his therapeutic performance and prescribe changes consistent with the broad limits of competence defined by the supervisor. In this way, supervision aims to help the clinician capitalize on his strengths and develop his own best individual therapeutic style. Although changes may involve personal philosophy, technical skill, or emotional understanding, emphasis is placed on the clinician's identification of problem behavior. Here the notion of clinical autonomy becomes more than a philosophy; it is a strategy of supervision.

Lewin (1951) has suggested that personal change involves "unfreezing" a person or group at their current operating level and inducing "movement" toward a new level of operation and refreezing at that new level. Although restraining forces and driving forces keep us in relative balance with our environment, restraining forces may be decreased and driving forces may be increased to induce unfreezing and movement. Unfortunately, conceptual frameworks involving clinician change have not yet been codified for use in speech pathology. We therefore must focus on the perceptions of the person to be changed. As supervisors, we must assess the clinician and client's driving and restraining forces and help induce movement toward new levels of operation. The major principles of behavioral change involve objectivity in perception, analysis of performance, and planned strategies for change. What the clinician intends to do (as evidenced in his lesson plan) is weighed against what he actually does in the therapy session and what the outcomes of his performance are (what the client says and does). Analysis in this context means systematically recording a range of behaviors which affect the therapeutic process and its outcomes.

Micro-therapy

Once the supervisor and clinician have proposed the necessary behavioral changes that the clinician is to realize in future therapeutic sessions, the component of micro-therapy may be included for training in discrete skills. The concept of micro-therapy is an outgrowth of micro-teaching and micro-counseling procedures widely used in the education and counseling professions. These procedures have imposing support for use in paraprofessional training (Haase and DiMattia, 1970), in teacher training (Rollin, 1970), in co-counseling supervision (Thielen, 1970), and in the training of medical students (Moreland, Ivey, and Phillips, 1973). Micro-therapy sessions are scaled-down, simulated therapy situations in which a student clinician and a volunteer client (usually another student clinician) role play therapeutic dialogue. During this mini-session, there is focused attention on the clinician's execution of a single therapeutic skill (for example, negative practice, negative reinforcement, intrapersonal monitoring, modeling, and so on). The single-skill concept is vital to training and is preferrable to teaching the clinician the entire array of therapeutic skills at once. Standard micro-therapy sessions consist of the following:

1. Videotaping of a 5-minute segment of micro-therapy between clinician and volunteer client.
2. Analysis and quantification of basal skill level.
3. Detailed instruction and demonstration of the therapeutic skill to be acquired. Videotaped models of the supervisor may be played for demonstration purposes.
4. A second 5-minute videotaped micro-therapy session between clinician and volunteer client.
5. Reanalysis and quantification of skill level achieved.
6. Retraining on a new skill or recycling back to step 3, depending upon skill level attained.

Micro-therapy training is best achieved in a group supervisory context. Multilevel instruction is employed by the supervisor and includes didactic instruction, demonstration, video-playback self-confrontation, and analysis. Perhaps the most important aspect of micro-therapy is the application of structured, focused feedback. Indeed, structured feedback is the basis for the phenomenon of learning itself. Students participating in micro-therapy have found it to be an important and valuable bridge to therapeutic practice.

CYCLE OF SUPERVISION

The basic method of this integrated supervisory process involves systematic, rational study and analysis of the clinician's behavior in therapy. Based on this study, supervisory procedures are implemented in order to enhance clinician development. These procedures aim to induce clinicians to think about, study, and analyze their clinical behavior and level of clinical development. The most productive way to enable clinicians to change their behavior is to involve them in the analysis of therapy. The clinician's focus should be on three major areas: 1) careful appraisal of his current behavior in relation to his ideal behavioral objectives, 2) the consideration of obstacles, both personal and technical, and 3), revised ways of thinking and behaving in the therapeutic situation. By the structure of the training cycle, the clinician can be led toward professional, autonomous development.

The supervisor and clinician learn to use the process together, in a joint effort whose aim is clinician development. Figure 6 illustrates the cycle of supervision in a systems analysis framework divided into three discrete phases: input, process, and output.

Input

The cycle itself begins with the input phase, where the clinician is engaged in therapy (step 1). Together the supervisor and clinician agree upon the selection of media that will be used to capture the events of therapy. After the therapy session, a supervisory conference is planned (step 2) in which the supervisor interacts in such a way that the clinician is led to scrutinize and explore his clinical behavior, reveal pertinent clinical events, define problems, and develop significant strategies. The conferencing session is vital for three reasons. First, through clinical introspection the clinician is afforded an opportunity to gain an important subjective

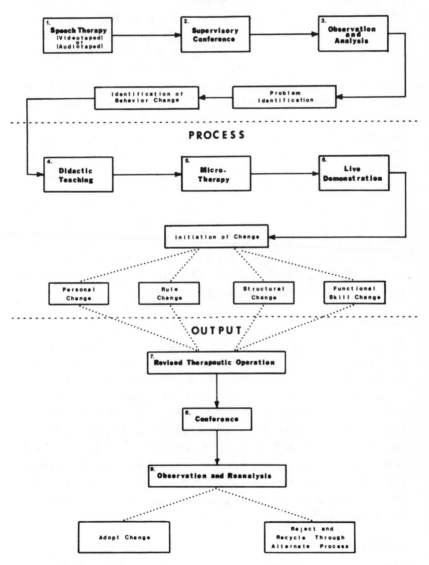

Figure 6. A systems analysis model of a comprehensive integrated supervisory process.

perspective on his practice, a perspective which is necessary for effective behavioral change. Second, the conference places the bulk of clinical decision making on the clinician, thus enhancing autonomy. Third, by way of the conference the supervisor develops insight into the clinician's subjective perceptions of the therapeutic process. This information enables the supervisor to structure supervisory operations accordingly. The supervisory conference is followed by the random selection of video- or audiotaped segments of therapy for objective observation and analysis (step 3). During the execution of these more objective procedures, the clinician's perceptions of problems and behaviors as revealed during the conference may be confirmed through means of quantification and analysis. After the analysis the supervisor and clinician jointly, or the clinician independently (depending upon his level of development), determine the clinician target behaviors which, because of their potential effect upon the client, should be changed or maintained.

Process

The process phase of the cycle involves three supervisory instructional elements: didactic teaching, micro-therapy, and demonstration. In this phase, the supervisor engages in one or more of these major elements (steps 4, 5, and 6 on Figure 6) which are designed to facilitate behavioral change. At this point, the supervisor must select and utilize the instructional procedure which is best suited to the clinician's independent needs. These procedures function to facilitate either personal changes, rule changes by which the clinician should operate, structural change within the therapy setting, or changes in functional skill level.

Output

Within the output phase of the model, based on the element of training, the clinician attempts to introduce the desired behavior changes into the future therapeutic session (step 7). Once again the supervisor and clinician engage in a post-therapy conference (step 8) followed by observation and reanalysis of therapy (step 9). At this point clinician and client target behaviors are compared with the previous analysis and with the criteria which have been set forth. Based on these data, the clinician behavior is either adopted or rejected, and then the clinician may be recycled through an alternate supervisory element to verify the attempted change.

SUMMARY AND COMMENTARY

Successful movement through the supervisory cycle requires that the supervisor employ his skill as a master clinician, skilled interactionist, and multi-resource person. Within the cycle of the integrated supervisory process are contained four types of training elements which can be summarized as:

1. Didactic teaching which results in information acquisition in keeping with current theory and research.
2. Specific and systematic observation and analysis which provide information relative to the clinician's and client's levels of therapeutic performance.
3. Performance exercises and instructional elements which facilitate clinical, behavioral change.
4. A context in which the supervisor communicates high level interaction to the student clinicians themselves, thus allowing for self-exploration and the emergence of the clinician's own idiosyncratic clinical self. Such communication enhances integration of technical knowledge with the clinioian's clinical skill, personal values, goals, and philosophy.

The model presented here raises many more questions than it answers. Considering the current status and time afforded supervision at most clinical training centers, the comprehensiveness of such an approach may be viewed as unrealistic. Nevertheless, the need to improve clinical training, coupled with the widespread endorsement of clinical supervision as a crucial component in the training of speech clinicians, warrants such as ideal worthy of being sought. It is time that we make a professional commitment to the status, practice, and research of clinical supervision.

REFERENCES CITED

Anderson, J. L., Supervision: The neglected component of our profession. In: J. L. Turton (ed.), Proceedings of a Workshop on Supervision in Speech Pathology. Ann Arbor: University of Michigan (1973).

Caracciolo, G. L., A model of clinical supervision based upon a Rogerian theoretical construct. Paper presented at the American Speech and Hearing Association convention, Houston (1976).

Cooper, M., Modern Techniques of Vocal Rehabilitation. Springfield, Ill.: Charles C Thomas (1973).

Culatta, R., A competency-based system for the initial training of speech pathologists. Asha, 18, 733–738 (1976).

Culatta, R., Colucci, S., and Wiggins, E., Clinical supervisors and trainees: Two views of a process. Asha, 17, 152–157 (1975).

Culatta, R., and Seltzer, H., Content and sequence analysis of the supervisory session. Asha, 18, 8–12 (1976).

Emerick, L., and Hood, S. B., (eds.), The Client-Clinician Relationship. Springfield, Ill.: Charles C Thomas (1974).

Erickson, R., and Van Riper, C., Demonstration therapy in a university training program. Asha, 9, 33–35 (1967).

Haase, R., and DiMattia, D., The application of the micro-counseling paradigm to the training of support personnel in counseling. Couns. Educ. Sup., 10, 16–22 (1970).

Lewin, D., Field Theory in Social Science: Selected Theoretical Papers. New York: Harper (1951).

Moreland, J., Ivey, A., and Phillips, J., An evaluation of micro-counseling as an interviewing training tool. J. Clin. Consult. Psychol., 41, 294–300 (1973).

Rollin, S., The development and testing of a performance curriculum in human relations. Unpublished doctoral dissertation, Amherst: University of Massachusetts (1970).

Schriberg, L. D., Filley, F. S., Hayes, D. M., Kwaitkowski, J., Schatz, J. A., Simmons, K. M., and Smith, M. E. The Wisconsin procedures for the appraisal of clinical competence (W-Pace): Model and data. Asha, 17, 158–165 (1975).

Sheehan, J. G., and Martyn, M. M., Therapy as seen by stutterers. J. Speech Hear. Res., 14, 445 (1971).

Sherif, M., and Sherif, C. W., Social Psychology. New York: Harper & Row (1969).

Thielen, T., The immediate effects of an abbreviated co-counseling supervision approach in teaching empathic skills to counselors in training. Unpublished doctoral dissertation, Bloomington: Indiana University (1970).

Index

American Speech and Hearing
  Association, 10
Analysis
  as behavioral change, 135–136
  as supervisory function, 8, 10
Analysis of Behavior of Clinicians
  System, 57
Analysis Sheet, 114–115
Authority figure in supervision,
  14
Autonomy, clinical, effected by
  supervision, 12

Behavior
  differences between exper-
    ienced and inexperienced
    clinicians, 61–65
  novel interactive, 100
  supervisor-clinician, defining,
    111–112
  supervisory, research on per-
    ception of, 77–82
Behavioral change, effected by
  supervision, 12
Boone-Prescott Interaction
  Analysis System, 57, 83

Certificate of Clinical Competence, 88
Client, interrelationship with
  supervisor and clinician, 9
Clinician
  becoming a, 33
  effective, 45–46
  fears held by, 34–36
  interrelationship with super-
    visor and client, 9
  as a person, 85–87
  and the therapeutic process,
    33–74
Clinics, weaknesses in supervisory
  procedures in, 5
Cognitive-didactic approach to
  supervisor-supervisee relationship, 12

Cognitive flexibility, 49
Communication as supervisory
  function, 8
Communication theorists, 76
Communicative atmosphere of
  conference, 99
Computer programming in
  analysis of clinical behavior,
  2
Conceptualization, universally
  accepted, of supervision, 13
Concreteness
  in clinician, 49
  in supervisory transactional
    system, 102–103
Conferences
  effective and ineffective, 81
  sample, 115–119
  support for supervision from, 2
  in client-centered supervision,
    18
  post-therapy, 133–134
Confidence in clinician, 49–50
Counseling
  in supervisory process, 13
  supportive, 110–111
Critique in supervision, 14

Delimiting factors in supervisory
  transactional system,
  108–109
Demonstration in supervision, 14
Directions, establishment of by
  supervisor, 8
Dyad
  interpersonal, 45, 98
  therapeutic, 45

Education
  models of supervision in, 13
  self-confrontation procedures,
    61
Effectiveness Rating Scale, 80
Empathy in supervisory transactional system, 100–101

145